100 Days Of Action: Build Your Online Nursing Business

DR. CATIE HARRIS

ISBN-13: 978-0-9982519-9-8

DEDICATION

This book was made possible through the encouragement of the dedicated nurses I work with every day in business as well as to Matthew who is my heart in everything I do.

CONTENTS

INTRODUCTION

The decision to start a business is something that should not be taken lightly. Contrary to public perception, starting a business is not fast nor easy. Sure there are some businesses that explode from day 1, but those are few and far between. You should expect to spend the first year of your business learning how to put together a business.

What I encourage my students to do is to anticipate a learning curve. As nurses, we have the expertise to start a business, but not the expertise of running the business. This isn't a major failing or reason not to start a business. In fact is most people don't know how to run a business when they get started.

As nurses we have this massive knowledge base of medicine, science, psychology, and the art and science of nursing. We have extensive education, certifications, licenses and degrees. Many of nurses are guilty of collecting an alphabet soup of letters behind their names in an attempt to "prove" something. I am certainly guilty of this. In fact I can't keep track of all my letters and now that I am in business they are almost irrelevant to me. Why? Because no one really cares about them. Yes, people are impressed by my PhD and the MBA. And people are shocked that I have 3 master's degrees in nursing, but none of it explains my success in business.

In fact, none of my degrees helped me start any of my businesses. When I finally invested in a mentor, we spent most of our time together helping me to unlearn my formal education because it was holding me back, not helping.

Now when I see nurses who want to start a business but don't do it because they need to "get certified as a health coach or a in a nutrition program or as a specialty nurse", it makes me crazy. Nurses are the most overeducated and over-experienced and least represented profession in entrepreneurialism.

Look, 20 year old entrepreneurs are sharing their "experience" and helping people to transform their lives for a lot of money. People with no professional expertise, no life experience and no credentials are self-proclaimed gurus. Health coaches are the biggest growing segment of entrepreneurialism. The opportunity for nurses to lead the way in this field is huge and wide open. And you don't need any more certifications.

What you need to do is STOP getting certifications and more degrees. Entrepreneurs are do-ers. Getting more certifications and degrees is a perfect example of procrastinating to the umpth degree.

You are good enough as you are right now. You can help people with what you already know today. You can easily put your knowledge and expertise into a business model. The only thing you are missing is the blueprint for setting your business up and getting clients.

I spent over $80,000 to learn from some of the biggest names in the industry in business, sales and marketing. I have incorporated this knowledge in my courses, books and emails. In fact in the summer of 2018, I wrote a blog series for my email subscribers called 100 Days of Summer. I wanted to provide them with the framework for how to put all the pieces of an online presence.

And it was A LOT!

I was surprised by the sheer amount of information that came out of that email series and about three quarters of the way through the summer I realized that I didn't just provide amazing value for my email readers → I wrote a book!

Literally, 100 emails = 200+ page book. This book that you are reading right now. Yes I needed to spruce it up a little bit and make some edits, but it was done over time. In fact 1 email a day equated to final project. This book is way better because I didn't recognize that I was writing a book until I was almost complete with the project. I was able to spruce it up, make it flow better and add a true purpose to the challenge.

This is a major concept that I like to promote to my students as well → doing 1 thing once a day is more productive than binge working on your business. You see, it's just as easy to burn out on your business as it is to burn out if you work too much at the hospital. You need to pace yourself.

There will always be more work to do at the hospital and in your business. But when you schedule your work, you schedule that 1 thing that needs to get done, it's 100x more likely that you will actually do it.

Think about it. Imagine you have a list of 50 things to do for your business to be successful or 1 thing to do. Clearly it's a no-brainer. But what most people don't get is that over time, doing one thing a day is more effective than having a list of 50 things to do. At least with 1 thing to do, and 1 thing to accomplish you can give your mind something it desperately seeks → instant gratification.

Your brain wants that short, easy win. That's why it's easy to do simple tasks, but you never seem to be able to get around to large, complex tasks.

The beauty of this book is that I have broken down your large, complex task of starting a business and creating an online presence into simple tasks that can be completed 1 day at a time.

In fact, give me 100 days and I will give you all the elements you need to setup your online presence for your nurse business.

Take it one day at a time, 1 thing at a time and be amazed at the progress you will make!

BLOGGING SUCCESS

Day 1 – Find Your Purpose

Several years ago, I read a blog called the Minimalists, and they said in one of their posts anyone could start a blog. Shortly thereafter I had this brilliant idea that I should start a blog.

It's easy they said.

They had step-by-step instructions.

I followed the instructions.

Sure enough in a few easy clicks I had a blog!

But now what?

There seemed to be a few steps missing between starting the blog and becoming an Influencer who makes millions of dollars living off endorsements and traveling the world.

Given I was about the 4,632,542nd blog to be created (I don't really know that for sure..), I felt like I was at a slight disadvantage.

Everyone had their opinion about what I should do next - set up a magazine blog, set up a sales blog, set up a non-magazine blog, get advertisers, don't get advertisers.

I spent a lot of time and a lot of money trying to figure out what to do with my blog, and now feel like I can share some very valuable insights with you.

The first thing you want to do is be clear about the purpose of your blog because everything that happens afterwards depends on this decision.

There are 3 broad reasons to start a blog and they are:

1. A blog to express yourself.
2. A blog that monetizes is generally a blog full of advertisers or affiliate marketing.
3. A blog for content marketing, which basically means to bring more traffic to your business website.

Action – Choose your reason for starting a blog.

Day 2 – Find Your Blogging Style

I told you there are 3 broad reasons to start a blog - to express yourself, to monetize and for content marketing. Let's dig a little deeper.

A blog to express yourself - This type of blog is where you share your thoughts and creative process with the world, kind of like an online diary. Your personal blog can be just for you or you can write for others, but generally without any intention to monetize or become Internet famous. Of course some people will make money or become famous, but most don't. This is generally where lifestyle blogs end up as well. Of course some people become famous, unfortunately millions more do not. So if you just want an online diary, you can set your blog up any way that you want.

The majority of bloggers want to do one of two things - either monetize directly from the blog or use it for content marketing. Since both of these are big topics to tackle, I'll talk about a blog that monetizes now and content marketing the next day.

How do you monetize a blog? Here are 4 ways to consider:

1. High traffic blogs such as WebMD or Mashable produce a TON of content and then sell space to advertisers. Every time someone comes to the blog and/or clicks on an ad, the owner makes money. In order to get sponsors to pay you for ads, you need a LOT of traffic. In order to get a lot of traffic, you need a lot of content. In order to get a lot of content, you need to write a lot of blogs - daily, ideally several times daily. This type of model was much easier to start several years ago, but still possible. You will need a strong plan for posting and a fierce determination to stick with it. Remember the high traffic blogs tend to have a team of writers who simply write all day long.

2. Write for a specific audience and build up your SEO (search engine optimization) with keywords. When visitors come to your site you sell products & services directly from your website.

3. You can also blog about products and services that other people sell and get paid through affiliate marketing. A great example of this type of blog is http://www.toptenreviews.com. Literally everything in this blog links to a product that if a visitor buys, then the owner gets paid a commission. Amazon has a similar affiliation program.

You could do product review blog posts and make money from commissions. With Amazon, if you send someone to their site to buy a particular item but the person doesn't buy that item you don't make a commission obviously. What most people don't know, however, is that if that person stays on Amazon's website and purchases anything else, you receive the credit for that sale. It's a pretty good deal! And one of the reasons Amazon has taken over the world…

4. Appeal to a large audience. Once you have over 100,000 fans, brands will begin to become interested in your influential power and will pay you to mention them in your posts or to share images and videos of you using their stuff. You will need to create raving fans by being authentic and genuine and likely sharing yoru daily life and experiences. A good example of someone making a living this way is Nas Daily. He creates 1 video that is 1 minute long every day.

The most common reason for starting a blog - content marketing is what we will talk about next.

Action – Decide if either of these options are right for your blog.

Day 3 – Content Is King

Content marketing is much different from a personal blog or a professional blog whose sole purpose is to monetize.

With content marketing, you don't need to write as much or often. You really just need to write some key articles and include some elements in each of your blog posts.

Let's start with the answer to the question of "what is content marketing?" Content marketing is writing specific content for your target audience with the intent of driving traffic to your website. If you own a business, it might be a really good idea for you to start a business blog.

You would write about the questions your target audience has that your product or service offers a solution. It's a great way to sell without selling. If someone "finds" you, you are actually a much more credible source then if you go searching for your audience via advertising to buy from you.

For instance, I write blog posts around the concept of nurses starting a business, so if a nurse types in "start a nurse business" in a Google search, my blog will likely come up on page 1. This makes me money because after reading my blog post, many nurses will search around my page and buy my products or services.

I don't have to write daily, weekly or even monthly. I add blog posts when I feel like it because the heavy work of my blog is already optimizing SEO (search engine optimization) and bringing nurses to my site. You only need a couple strong blog posts which can carry you on page 1 of Google for years to come.

Content marketing is highly recommended for any business you start or even if you just want to amass an audience.

Tomorrow I will tell you exactly how to figure out what your target audience is searching for so you can begin content marketing.

Action – Decide if you want to do content marketing.

Day 4 – The Secrets Of Mankind

There is one place where the deepest darkest secrets of mankind are told. There is basically nothing that isn't asked or revealed in this one place.

And that place is Google.

If you want to know the answer to something, what do you do? You Google it of course. So what if you could look over the shoulder of your audience and see exactly what they are typing into Google? Why would this be helpful? It would be helpful, because whatever comes up on the first page of Google are the links that person is going to follow. In fact over 95% of Google searches stop on page 1.

99% of Google searches end on page 2. This means if you aren't coming up on page 1 of Google when your audience is looking for information on your topic, then your content marketing isn't SEO optimized. One of the ways you can optimize your SEO is through ranking for keywords. Keywords are the "words" people use to search for the answer to a problem.

For instance, if I need a plumber in Philadelphia, I would type in "plumbers in Philadelphia". If I wanted Tai Chi classes, I would type in "Tai Chi in Philadelphia". If you owned a Tai Chi facility, you would want to rank for these keywords exactly. Maybe you could write a blog post called "The Best Tai Chi Classes in Philadelphia". Now if you are a nationwide service, this wouldn't necessarily work, but roll with me here for a second.

This is how your content marketing works and it's free.

You can buy Google ads to come up on page 1, but this has gotten extremely expensive and competitive. You couldn't afford to rank for a keyword like "nursing". The competition on that word is so fierce you would spend $80 every time someone clicked on your ad.

Let's go back to keywords for a moment. Before you start content marketing the first thing you need to do is find the keywords your audience is Googling because you want to write a killer blog post using a keyword or phrase that you want to rank for.
One of the best ways to find keywords is to open up the Google Keyword

Tool in Adwords. Here are the steps:

1. Open an Adwords account. (you need a gmail account to open Adwords)
2. Sign up for Adwords. It's free, but you have to put in all your information
3. Once you are signed up, Adwords forces you to set up an ad. Go through the motions of setting up an ad. I'm not sure why you have to do this, but you do in order to get to the Keyword Tool
4. After you set up an ad (make sure it's not running!!!), go to the top of the search bar. You will see 4 Headlines: Home - Campaigns - Opportunities - Tools
5. Hover over Tools and you'll see Keyword Tool
6. Play with a variety of words and terms that you think your audience would use to Google a solution that you provide. The Keyword Tool will actually let you know if people really are searching with that term or if there is a better term you could rank for.

Pro Tip: Go for keywords that have good volume (1k-100k/month) but have a low cost. You don't want to try to rank for the word "nurse" or "breast cancer". This would be extremely expensive. The prices you see are per click.

Another free option is to use the Keyword Tool Dominator. You can search 3 free keywords a day on this tool, which will give you incredibly valuable info. Or you can purchase it for $39.99 to do unlimited searches. You get the same information from a free Adwords account, so I would recommend doing that first.

Find 5 keywords/phrases you want to rank for in Google and tomorrow I'll give you 5 ways to optimize your SEO (search engine optimization).

You want to do all of this BEFORE starting your blog. Planning will save you a lot of time...

Action – Find 5 keywords or phrases to rank for in the Adwords Keyword Tool.

Day 5 – Search Engine Optimization

Maybe you've heard of SEO in the past and didn't really get what it was about. Search Engine Optimization (SEO) is a ranking system. How you rank when someone is searching for a keyword is vital to content marketing.

For instance, if I want to know what a paleo diet is, whoever has the best SEO is going to be the website that Google shows me first and typically the one I go to.

Most searches end with page 1 of Google, so if you aren't on page 1 you are missing out on this huge free marketing advantage. Plus the value of being found as opposed to direct advertising cannot be understated. This is a huge advantage!

You can build in SEO into your blogs before you write them so they work hard to get you clients or to bring an audience to your website.

Here are 5 ways to optimize your blog for SEO using the keywords you chose to rank for.

1. Put the keyword in the title of your blog
2. Put the keyword in the headline of your blog post
3. Put the keyword in the image of your blog
4. Use the keyword in the first 100 words of your blog post
5. Add the keyword to the permalink of the URL

Have no idea what that means? Over the next couple of days, I'll explain each one of these SEO strategies, which will bring you fame and fortune if you use them correctly!

Action – Do a search of your competition. See who is ranking on page 1 of Google using the keywords or phrases you want to rank for.

Day 6 – Driving Traffic

In order to optimize SEO of your blog to drive more traffic to your website, there are 5 locations that you need to place your keywords. Remember, we are creating our first blog post, using one of the keywords or phrases that we found by using the Google Keyword Tool.

Once we have the keyword that we want to rank for, we are going to place that keyword in 5 distinct locations to optimize SEO.

Writing for a blog is unlike any academic assignment you've ever had. First, unlike your college research course, we are going to write the title of our blog post first.

We need to make sure we get our keyword or phrase into the title so that it makes sense.

Let's take my student Lori as an example. Lori is a writing coach for DNP students. She teaches them to write scholarly projects and graduate.

One of her keywords terms might be: "Help With DNP Project". According to Google, it's not a massively high volume search (this is a niche area), but sufficient numbers of nurses are looking for help with their DNP project and this is what they are asking Google to show them.

To optimize SEO and to rank high on this topic, Lori could title her first blog:

10 Tips To Help Nurses Write The DNP Project

Or some variation of that. The term doesn't have to be exact, but really close is good.

Now that the title is written, you need to outline the blog post using headlines. What are the 3-5 major points you want to convey in this blog post? Make these the headlines.

Headlines are helpful to Google to determine if your blog is what the end user is looking for. If your headlines have the keyword, Google will rank your post higher than others.

Find a way to make sure the keyword term is included in one of them. In Lori's case her 3 headlines could be:

1. Struggling with the DNP Project Idea
2. Brainstorming the DNP Project
3. How to write the DNP project

Also make sure the keyword is used within the first 100 words of the post.

Optimizing for SEO doesn't make sense for every single blog post, but it's important to write specifically for SEO for several of your blog posts. SEO can take several weeks to take effect, so get these blog posts written first.

There is no magic number, but 5 SEO blog posts would be a great goal to have. Try writing out 5 Titles using your keywords. We'll figure out what to write in the blog post later.

We still have 2 more places to optimize SEO in our blog post, which is coming tomorrow.

Action – Using the keyword you want to rank for, create a title for your first blog post, and outline 3-5 headlines that have the keyword in them. Write the first 100 words with the keyword in that paragraph.

Day 7 – Still Optimizing

Images carry a lot of weight in the Google algorithm – which is how Google decides which content to show. It's not random! Make sure you use images in your blog post.

A side note, please do not take any old image off the Internet, there are copyright laws that you need to abide by. Either purchase the credit to use stock photo or use websites that allow you download pictures for use on your blog. A couple sites are Unsplash.com, Pexels.com and Pixabay.com

The next thing you want to do is to rename the property of the photo using your keywords. If you upload the image to your blog on your website, make sure you rename the file as the keyword. This is a fast and easy way to optimize SEO. Don't miss this step, it's like a critical freebie!

The last way to optimize your blog SEO is to change the slug or permalink to include the keyword. Most websites will allow you customize the slug. For instance, my website is CatieHarris.com. My blog site is: CatieHarris.com/blog.

If I wrote a blog on Nurses in Business, the URL may be:

CatieHarris.com/blog/**2018Havslkfowieofj**

The bolded part of the URL is the permalink or slug. You can change that and be sure to rename it with your keyword. Once I make the change, the new URL would be:

CatieHarris.com/blog/**nursesinbusiness**

Again, a real fast and easy way to optimize SEO that you shouldn't miss!

Action – Add an image to your blog post and change the name of the image to include your keyword. Change the permalink (slug) to the keyword when you post the blog to your website.

Day 8 – Write Like You Talk

A blog post is not scholarly writing, it's not a dissertation and it's not hard. Write like you talk. Don't clean it up in "professional" language. Your post needs to be easy to read and your point needs to be clear and concise. In fact, have your kids read it. If they have no idea what you are talking about, rip it up and start over.

Aim for 300-500 words, this is about half a page to a page. That is more than enough.

Generally start off your blog post with a problem, issue or insight. Just ONE problem, issue or insight. Not 2 or 3, or 10.

The body can be research, proof, testimonials or your argument. The last part of your blog is a summary of your main point and your call to action.

Make sure you always ask your reader to do something such as "leave a comment", "Like my page", "read this interesting post", "download my free guide".

Use this structure over and over for best results!

Tomorrow, I will teach you how to never run out of ideas of what to write.

Action – Get your first blog post written and SEO optimized

Day 9 – Never Run Out Of Ideas

Returning to my student Lori who is the DNP Coach, she can write her initial SEO blog on 10 Tips To Help Nurses Write The DNP Project.

Then she is free to write other posts. But what to write about? Lori can continue to write on the same topic from various different angles. She no longer needs to be as diligent with SEO titles and headlines, because she has a couple posts that are already optimized. The thing is sometimes titles don't make sense when they are SEO optimized. Don't stress on that. A couple SEO optimized posts are sufficient.

She can still optimize the images and the permalinks (slugs). I would encourage everyone to do that.

At first glance, Lori might think she has said all there is to say on a topic, but that couldn't be any further from the truth. There are literally 20 different blog posts that could come from the one topic that she wrote about.

It's not a one and done deal where you write once on a topic and then you are through with it. Lori should write a lot of variations on the same topics.

She could do a case study story about one her students and how she helped them with their DNP Project.

She could write a review of books on DNP projects. She could evaluate the best DNP programs or faculty. She could interview faculty on their strengths. She could write about why students need help, how a mentor could help, mistakes students make without help, why it's better to do it right the first time, time management… etc

Don't be afraid to write the same concept over and over again, just tweak it for different audiences. Remember once it's a blog, it's a vlog, a social media post, an email, etc. Repurpose all your content. You don't have to do it all at once, but remember to come back to it.

Maybe you get the point right? This can be super easy. It doesn't need to be a monstrous project. Many blog posts are 300-500 words. In fact, you don't want most of your blog posts to be too long. Short, to the point, clear about one thing.

But this isn't the hardest part about blogging, I'll tell you what is tomorrow...

Action – Come up with 5-10 blog ideas based on your keyword and audience interests.

Day 10 – The Hardest Thing

The hardest part about blogging is committing to doing it. Your initial enthusiasm may help you to write a few blogs, and if they are SEO optimized, that may just be enough.

You don't need to blog every day, unless you have made a commitment to do so or you are trying to monetize the blog. If your blog is for content marketing than having 10 great blog posts could be all you ever need.

Not every blog needs hundreds of posts. Honestly a blog with too many posts may be overwhelming and scare people away. Make sure you organize your blog posts with categories and tags so readers can easily find posts that would interest them.

Don't expect your audience to scroll through 10 pages of blogs looking for something of interest to them. Be a good host and make it easy.

If you want to blog on a regular basis to build up a loyal following, I would suggest setting up an editorial calendar and setting deadlines for yourself. Make a plan to blog on a consistent basis. It could be monthly, weekly, daily, whatever, but stick to your choice for at least 6 months. Having this consistency will help your readers trust you

Ok, ok, so now you have a blog, where do you put these blog posts? Tomorrow starts our journey through websites and beyond.

Whether you want to know what your free options for a website are or you are ready to spend lots of money for customization, I'll tell you what you can expect and how to get started.

Action – Set up an editorial calendar for how frequently you are going to write blog posts.

WEBSITES 101

Day 11 – The Personal Website

Now that you have your blog(s) written (or you plan to write them soon!), you need a place to put them. There are so many options out there it can be a little overwhelming. There are social media platforms, free website platforms, semi-customized website platforms, shopping website platforms. How are you supposed to pick the right one?

Well if you know why you are writing a blog then this decision is easier.

If you blog is simply for personal use - stick with free social media platforms or free website platforms like Wordpress.com or Tumblr. You can also use social media as a place to post your blogs as well. You could post on LinkedIn or Facebook. You could even do stories on Instagram or put together Pinterest pictures. You could post in any format – images, videos, blogs, etc.

However, it's difficult to monetize or sell on social media, so those aren't the best choices if you want to monetize a blog. Social media is for social gatherings. If you want to monetize a blog such as doing product reviews or selling arts and crafts, you might consider opening a blog on Shopify or Etsy and using the blog to drive traffic straight to your marketplace.

If you are looking to compliment your business with a blog, then there are few more things to consider. For the sake of simplicity, I am going to assume everyone wants to complement their website with the blog, so we will talk about which type of websites would be appropriate for this category tomorrow.

Action – Determine if you are creating a personal website or professional.

Day 12 – A Social Media Website

Your business can exist solely on social media and many social media stars do this. You can blog on Facebook or LinkedIn or do vlog (video blogs) on You Tube. You could even just post pictures on Pinterest and Instagram and cultivate a following. It really all just depends on you and how you like to communicate.

Many business owners, however will use social media as a way to disseminate a blog and not the only place to house it. Think of social media as the extension of your blog. Every time you post a blog on your website, you can post a link to it on LinkedIn, Twitter, Facebook, or whatever platforms you are on. You can even pick out a highlight from your blog and create a quick vlog to upload onto You Tube.

One quick and easy way to do this is to set up a social media manager such as Hootsuite. Hootsuite has a very useful free version that will let you schedule posts and links to all your social media accounts just through using their dashboard. This way you don't need to sign into each platform separately. You can manage them all through Hootsuite.

Hootsuite also lets you set up streams so you can follow certain hashtags or conversations or what your competitors are talking about.

Pretty nifty!

There are limits to the free version of course, but you can set up at least 3 accounts and it's 3 less accounts you need to worry about maintaining. Even if you use a separate website for your blogs, but have social media accounts, this service is worth investigating.

Action – Determine which social media accounts you are going to post to and set up a free Hootsuite account.

Day 13 – Should You Get A Wordpress Website?

More than 70% of websites are built on Wordpress.org (Not wordpress.ORG is different from wordpress.COM, I know it's confusing). That's pretty impressive. Does that mean you should be too?

Well Beginner Beware..

Yes setting up a wordpress.org website with one click is super easy and yes it is completely 100% customizable. But…. once you set up the website with one click, it looks nothing like a real website.

You will then be immersed into a world of widgets, plugins and figuring out frameworks, child frameworks and buying one that you want.
This is also easy enough, however, in order to get a framework to look the way you want, you will need to understand HTML and CSS.

You can use the pre-build frameworks that Wordpress has installed, but you still need to learn all the widgets and plugins. Expect to spend several weeks figuring it out. In fact, wordpress.org has a massive tutorial space where you can spend a couple weeks immersed in learning all about it.

Wordpress.org is amazing and it's extremely powerful, but is it what you need?

To get wordpress.org to the level you want it will cost $750-1000 to get a rigid framework set up. A semi-customized site will cost you about $3000-5000 and a fully customized site will start at $10,000.

What are your other options? I'll give you a few starting tomorrow

Action – Check out wordpress.ORG and some of it's reviews

Day 14 – Rigid Websites

A rigid website is one that has limited options. While this might not sound great, it is good for people who know nothing about coding or websites as well as for people who want to know nothing about coding or websites. A website platform like Wix or GoDaddy are very rigid. They have drag and drop capability. Which is great because you literally just change words and images and you are done.

What's not great is when you want to do something slightly different than what is available on the platform. Just forget about it. If you don't like exactly what you see, there isn't much that can be done differently on these websites.

Does that matter? Well if you talk to website designers they will tell you it's the difference between a so-so business and a killer business. After several years of doing websites, I now believe that is a bunch of hype and nonsense to get you to pay extraordinary fees.

Christy D'Arcy from CityHydration.com set up on Wix.com and she has no problem getting business. I know people who have spent $10,000 on a website and can't make a dime.

Now if you are the type who obsesses over the perfect website, then a rigid website is not for you. If you want something cheap and easy and you're not concerned about email marketing or the latest trends in website development and marketing, then here are a couple options:

GoDaddy costs about $9 a month and Wix will cost between $15-20/month.

A good deal? Maybe. Having any website up and running is better than no website. If you are just starting out and you don't have a budget at all for websites or the time to learn HTML/CSS, then these might be a good choice. You will likely grow out of your website quickly, but at these prices it's a good deal. Which do I recommend? Stay tuned.

Action – Check out GoDaddy and Wix.com websites. Don't buy anything yet, let's explore your options.

Day 15 – Semi-Customized Websites

Remember I told you semi-customized wordpress.org sites start around $3000 to have built for you? Well here is another option and the option I love that is super cheap - Squarespace. Squarespace allows you build extremely professional semi-customized websites that integrate with a variety of apps. This is a big deal, such as scheduling apps, commerce apps, and all different functions. Take a look.

You can do just about anything on Squarespace like podcasts, videos, blogs, sell products and services, build out optins, newsletters and even an RSS feed. The important thing about Squarespace is that you can grow with it. As you learn more about email marketing and website development you can expand your Squarespace site. Squarespace is also fully optimized and gets preferential treatment in Google algorithms, meaning all things the same, you will rank higher. Oftentimes Google will ignore rigid websites regardless of how great your content is.

Squarespace will cost you around $15 a month. If you want to set up a store with commerce it's more expensive (and unnecessary, I would recommend running all your commerce through Paypal).

You can use it like a rigid website and just change out images and texts or you can use the functions they have to rearrange templates and add in features. You can even hire a coder to make it 75% customizable, but this is completely unnecessary. There is a little bit of a learning curve with Squarespace, so I recommend you watch their tutorials.

If you purchase an annual subscription, you will even get your domain name for free and a year's worth of G-suite, which includes a domain specific email - A MUST for any business. So if you domain name is SusieQ.com, then your domain specific email could be: info@susieq.com. This is much better than susieq1234@gmail.com.

Squarespace is definitely worth a look.

Action – Go to Squarespace and look at the gorgeous, professional templates they have. Compare them to GoDaddy and Wix.

Day 16 – Fully Loaded Websites

If you want to go all out and get your website fully customized and optimized for your business, expect to pay about $10,000 to start. You will have a gorgeous website on wordpress.org, but don't do it yourself. If you can't afford the cost, stick with one of the other types of websites.

A designer should set up your website so it's optimized to convert prospects who come to your website into customers. In a couple days, I'll give you how to do this for a lot less.

When you have the funds for a fully customizable site wordpress.org would be advisable. This is a huge expense and not a good move for a business that is just starting out. This might be a goal you aim for in the future.

Action – See if you tell the difference between a $10k website and DIY Squarespace website.

Day 17 – Shopping Websites

Now there are specialty types of websites that you might consider. For instance if you are just going to sell products, it might more sense for you to build your website completely on a Shopify store.

You can blog in Shopify and do a host of other things, so it might be worth checking out. Same with an Etsy store, you can host everything right in their site. Just remember those platforms belong to Shopify and Etsy, so if they go out of business so do you! And if they don't like what you are doing, they can shut you down at any time. The cost of a shopping website is about the same as you would expect to pay for Squarespace or Wix.

The last type of website you can build that I want to tell you about is 22 social. 22 social is a website platform that is completely built off of Facebook. You won't even recognize you are on a Facebook platform when you use 22 social. Check out how 22 social has morphed these plain Facebook pages into semi-customized websites. If your audience is on Facebook, this might be a great option for you. Remember though, Facebook can and does change its rules all the time. You may need to constantly adapt your business or 22social page based on the change du jour.

Tomorrow I'll teach you how to design the perfect website no matter what platform you use.

Action – Check out 22social and see what those Facebook pages look like.

Day 18 – Website Templates: The Header

When you enter into a hospital unit, you expect to see certain things, a nursing station, some rooms, a hallway. The same is true of websites. Over the years, people have been conditioned to respond in certain ways to the layout of a website.

What was acceptable 10 years ago – putting as much information and color on a website as possible, is not good business. In fact if your website is a mess or not well organized, this can repel people. They will instantly jump off your site.

This includes having 100 advertisers or pop ups. If you put all kinds of detractors on your website people will run away as quickly as possible.

There is such thing as a perfect template for websites. It starts with the header. Your header should be an image that reflects what you do. It should make sense. It should have 1 headline that tells people who come to your page EXACTLY what you do.

You don't want to be cute or clever here. For instance if I go to an auto insurance website, I don't want to see a mountain and a headline that says "Be one with your car". I want to know if they sell auto insurance and how much.

Ideally in this case the header would be an image of a smiling person next to a car and the headline says "We sell car insurance at great rates". This is an excellent header.

When someone comes to your website, the first thing they see is the header. This is prime real estate. So why do so many people waste this space? They put pretty pictures or videos up, that look cool, but they don't convert prospects into customers. In fact they are confusing to people. They wonder why they are on your site and quickly bounce.

For example, if you are a coach and you teach diabetics how to live a healthy life, you could have a picture of a happy woman making a healthy meal. Your header title might read: Reduce your Blood Sugar in 90 days eating delicious and healthy food.

Think about what transformation you provide for your clients and then make that the header. When a visitor comes to your website they will see what outcome you specialize in and they will see happy people. This is actually quite powerful. Look at websites the next time you are surfing and see which ones draw you in.

Action – Choose your website platform and create a header for your website.

Day 19 – The Optin

What comes after the header on your website? It should be your opt-in.

What's an opt-in? An opt-in is something free you offer your audience in exchange for their email address. Think about what your audience would love to have. For instance, my student Lori is the DNP Coach. She offers free templates for DNP students to structure their capstones.

What does she do with their email addresses? She sends them a weekly email update on things of interest to DNP students. How does she make money? Well if a DNP student needs a writing coach or some editing work, all she needs to do is contact Lori. After all Lori has already established a relationship with that DNP candidate through her weekly emails.

More on email marketing later…

Action – Make sure whichever platform you choose allows you to add in an opt-in form.

Day 20 – About You

Finally the last part of your website should be about you and your services. Who are you and what do you offer? Make sure your "About Me" section isn't all about you. Yes, I know that sounds weird, but your About Me section should be about your audience. So yes, you tell your story but in a way that your audience can relate to.

If your business is about COPD patients, there must be a reason why you started it. Maybe you have worked with COPD patients for years, or you had a family member who suffered, or you see people suffering with COPD. Whatever the reason, you want to make sure the person with COPD who comes to your website is nodding their head, like yeah, this person gets me, they understand my struggles and they have an answer for me.

If someone believes you understand them, they will naturally believe that you can help them as well.

Once you complete your About Me section (add in a photo or video too!), then let people know how they can work with you. Do you offer 1:1 coaching, group coaching, online courses, an e-book etc? This section doesn't need to be long, maybe a couple paragraphs. Whatever it takes to get across to your audience that you understand them.

Next, I will teach you how to brand your website and company. This is much more important than picking out a logo. Branding is fundamental to pricing and positioning.

Action – Create an About Me section.

IT'S ALL IN THE BRAND

Day 21 – Branding 101

Branding is the fun part of business. At least for me. Who doesn't love picking out pretty colors and designing business cards? Sigh… if only these things were actually important and made any difference in my business.

Because unfortunately, in the early stages branding such as colors, logos and business cards are really not that important. Yet most people spend an inordinate amount of time choosing colors and creating business cards. I spent more time designing my business card then I did putting my business together.

There is one explanation for this behavior - Procrastination.

Pure and simple procrastination. It's easy, it's not taxing on your brain, and it actually does very little for you in the initial stages. The real branding is hard work and most people avoid it. I'll tell you about that over the next few days.

Yes, yes, I know we all want to do it right the first time and not have to deal with redoing the branding. But let it be said here first, if you spend more than an hour on all of your colors, fonts and logos, you're procrastinating…

Tomorrow, let's pick some colors and do some fun stuff.

Action – Finish up finalizing your website platform and working on your 1st SEO optimized blog posts.

Day 22 - Colors

Picking out colors is one of my favorite things to do! I could get lost on color wheels for hours. Choosing a color palette for your brand, is just, well so exciting.

The first thing I want you to do is check out this blog post by a designer that is perfect for what you need to know. Read this and then come back: https://tinyurl.com/nursepreneurcolor

Now the next thing you need to do is decide what you want your primary color to be for your brand. After reading the article above you should have some sense of what type of emotion you want to elicit for your audience. Please also remember to choose colors for your audience not because you like them! For instance, hot pink as a primary color might work for millennial girls, but not men and elderly people. You could however use a touch of pink in any design.

It's important to start with that primary color first. Then you can add in other colors that actually match. Let the color wheel help you.

One more thing before picking a color palette for your brand. Once you pick your brand colors, you need to stick with them. If you choose a navy color, you need to use the same navy color EVERY TIME. Not something that looks similar to the last navy you choose. Your eye may not be able to tell the difference, but subconsciously you can. Colors have code names and are identified as HEX numbers.

Copy the hex number of every color you choose. Then whenever you are in a different program you use that hex code to find your color. Again, don't pick random colors because you can't remember the hex code of your color palette. Keep that color palette on sticky notes and put them everywhere you need to reference them.

There are also different ways to identify colors such as RGB (red, green, blue hues), and HSI (which is a color saturation percentage). Different programs ask for different codes. Translating HEX to RGB or HSI is easy.

Take the HEX code and google how to convert that hex code to RGB and then to HSI percentages. Then put those codes somewhere that will be easy for you to find and reference quickly.

Now the fun part… Go to this website: https://coolors.co/, go to the top right and select: Generate. Then just choose your color palette. You can generate options or you can explore your own.

Use the spacebar on your computer to change the color palette. If you see a color you love, use your mouse and hover over the color. You will see a padlock. This will lock the color while you change the others. Go ahead and lock which color you want and then keep using the spacebar to find other colors that will match it.

Action – Choose your color palette for your brand

Day 23 - Fonts

Now I will tell you with certainty that I never knew how complicated font theory could be. I also had no idea of its impact on mood and emotion. I cannot do a good job explaining how this works so I'm sending you to an article on fonts instead.

Just know that your font matters. There are other fonts aside from Times New Roman and Ariel. Again when you are creating a personal or business brand you want consistency. Don't mix and match fonts based on whatever pops up on your computer program. If you choose to work in open sans you stay in open sans.

General rule of thumb, no more than 3 different types of fonts. Get in and get out of font world. Use something standard. If you choose a crazy font, you will have to download and upload it to every program you use. You may even need to pay to use the font if it's very unique, so choose wisely…

Check this article out: https://tinyurl.com/nursepreneurfont

Action – Choose your fonts for your brand.

Day 24 – Final Decisions

Ok, so today is the big day! You've chosen your colors and your fonts.

Congratulations! Remember you don't want to veer away from these colors and fonts. Of course you can grow out of them, or change them over time, just not on a daily basis or with every new blog post you write or every new article.

Above all you want consistency in your design. This is part of what branding is about. At the end of the day, you are creating a general feel. Colors and fonts can make people have different feelings. Kind of like when you open an email AND IT'S ALL IN CAPS AND IT MAKES YOU FEEL ANXIOUS.

The font and colors you choose will create a mood. Be aware and intentional about what you choose. Also remember to choose fonts that are readily available to you. Not all the same fonts are found in Word or Google docs or whatever program you are using, such as canva.com, etc. This will invariably add a level of frustration and annoyance if you are working in an obscure font or one you have to purchase and upload to every program.

Beware of procrastinating too much on this topic. Some of the variations in colors and fonts are so negligible, so if you are trying to decide among 3 or 4 options that look a little similar, just pick the one that is more common. Consistency over anything else is what truly matters.

Action – Make your final decision on your color palette and fonts.

Day 25 - Logos

Another fun day! Let's create your logo. Now one of the reasons we waited so long to create a logo is because you need to use your colors and fonts. You can't really choose your colors and fonts until you know what you are selling or who your audience is.

And you can't know who your audience is until you know what you are good at and what to do! This is why the whole topic of branding doesn't even come up in my signature NursePreneur Business Academy until almost 12 weeks into the program.

But if you already have a business or know exactly what you are going to sell then you can go forward with your logo.

You can have a logo designed by a place like 99designs.com or Fiverr.com. You'll get some basic designs that quite frankly will be good enough. You don't need a Picasso, just something that is consistent with what your company does and it retains the rest of your brand. Remember to use your fonts and colors in your logo!

Action – Check out Fiverr.com and 99designs.com to see if this is an option for you to get a logo created.

Day 26 – The DIY Option

Canva.com is a life-changer. I don't say this lightly but canva.com truly changed my life forever. I used to send every picture to my brother to resize for the most mundane and ridiculous things such as a Facebook post. Why he didn't just tell me to get Canva is beyond me. I did finally discover it and now my brother has started opening my emails again.

If you've ever struggled with images and designs, you will love Canva.

Canva allows you to create amazing designs on their platform on the image size you need. For instance if you want to create a Facebook banner, Canva gives you the pixel size and dimensions. You can design your banner without Facebook butchering it because your pixels were out of whack.

Now I don't want to go into all the amazing joys of Canva - you'll see for yourself, but there is the one feature I want to tell you about that is pertinent here and that is the logo creator. Choose a logo as a design option in canva and literally tons of predesigned logos come up for you. You simply change out the words and pictures and you are set!

I didn't even tell you the best part yet. Canva is completely FREE. There is a paid version, but I don't know anyone who actually uses it. Canva is so amazing in the free version, there is just no reason to upgrade.

Maybe poor planning on their part? I use Canva so much, I feel guilty and would like to pay them.. Check it out and create your own logo for free. www.Canva.com

Action – Check out canva.com

Day 27 – Images

One more thing before I tell you all about what real branding is… I just want to give you some resources for getting pictures online. Remember, you can't just take any old picture off the Internet. While that might fly when you are putting together a powerpoint for class, it won't work in the world of blogging or putting together a business.

There are literally companies who go around finding people using pictures illegally in their business just so they can penalize them. Don't do it. Don't make a habit of it.

You either need to set up an account with a Stock photo company and pay them the required licensing fees or buy the photo outright. There are royalty free sites where you can download pictures. Be careful though, because there are still some limitations of what you can and cannot do to these pictures, so be sure to read the licensing agreeement.

Royalty Free Images

- https://unsplash.com/
- https://www.pexels.com/
- https://stocksnap.io/
- http://picography.co/
- http://www.gratisography.com/
- https://picjumbo.com/
- https://500px.com/
- https://iso.500px.com/

My absolute favorite is unsplash.com.

Action – Check out the royalty free image sites

Day 28 – Packaging

Branding is all about the experience you provide for your audience. What do you offer? How do you offer it? Are you a Walmart brand or a Gucci brand? Everything plays a part in defining how you are perceived by your audience.

The first element in building a brand is how you package what you offer. What is it that you offer the world? What is your solution to a given problem?

On one end if your solution to being overweight is to diet, then your brand is pretty generic and non-specific. When you get to the next two elements - pricing and positioning - there will be very little you will be able to do to separate yourself from, well just about everyone else.

Yes, eating less and exercising more is the mathematical key to weight loss. However, this formula has been systematically unsuccessful in reducing obesity in the U.S. at least.

Maybe you have lost weight, or you have helped others to lose weight. Was it simply you ate less or was there a little more to it? Maybe you overcame adversity, you overcame some challenge - abuse, failure, loss, etc. If you can deconstruct the process of how you lost weight and can transfer that process to others, then you not only have a business, you have a unique brand. You can package this process into a system.

Why would you package the steps into a system? Because it gives you more credibility.

If you tell me to go lose 30 pounds by dieting, I'm not going to do it. More often than not it's too overwhelming. People shut down on the idea because they don't' know where to start or how to start. Now there are hundreds, if not thousands of weight loss programs, but there is always room for more. Why? Because people are still obese, and looking for the right system.

I recently found my weight loss guru. After years of yo-yo weight, I have kept it off with this woman's system. It spoke to me and I found I could follow it. She had a system, a method, a structure. I trusted her, I liked her brand. She gave me grocery lists, she told me what to do and I did it. And I lost weight!

Does it matter that there are 1 million ways of saying the same thing? No. Because sometimes people just need to hear it your way to make it work.

Now the great part of putting together a package is what you can do next…

Action – What is your system? If you don't have a system yet, you need to check out my course: Systematize Your Expertise on my website. Use this page for special pricing:
https://catieharris.com/systematize-your-expertise-special/

Day 29 - Pricing

Pricing is an element of business where everyone gets a little crazy. People tend to undercharge or overcharge by orders of magnitude. My student Erin was doing in-home personal training for an hour at 5am for $20 an hour. Whereas, I have another student who thinks she is worth $1000 an hour without providing any proof or substantiating the claim.

I'm sure your mom thinks your services are great, but there is an element of earning your respect in the marketplace and proving your system first. Here's the thing, when you are just starting out and you have very little credibility and you're a marketplace nobody, you just can't jump in and charge what other people are charging, but you don't want to charge way less either. If I see 5 coaches charging $100/hr and you are charging $20/hr, I don't think "Oh, what a great deal", I think "I wonder what's wrong with the coach who only charges $20/hr".

So you want to be conscientious about pricing. Don't under bid everyone. You're not Walmart!

Here is a good rule of thumb. When you are first starting out test your package on people - for FREE. You may even have to beg, plead and harass people to test your package out for free (basically because no one values information they get for free). Yes, for free, help them out, get transformations, get testimonials, get proof. Ironically it's harder to get results when you train for free, but it's a necessary evil.

Once you have these things, then you have earned the right to charge right smack in the middle of the group. Look at what your competitors are charging, and you charge the same. Then, when you have indisputable proof that your system or offering really works, you have media attention, then you can start raising your prices to wherever you want that people will still pay. Pricing will just be a series of testing until you have enough work at a price that you are happy with. That is the unscientific yet logical methodology of pricing yourself in the marketplace!

Action – What are your competitors charging for similar services or offerings?

Day 30 – Positioning

Positioning is the another part of branding that is extremely important to manage. Your position in the marketplace will be determined by your packaging and pricing. For instance, Walmart positions itself on price - something I would strongly discourage you from doing!

You as the consumer would expect to pay $20 for a handbag at Walmart. You do not go there looking for a $2000 Gucci bag or some Tiffany diamonds.

When you go to the Gucci store, you don't ask them for their $20 selection. You expect to pay a lot of money when you go there. That is their positioning. A big part of positioning is the experience the client undergoes while in your world.
If I go to Gucci and know I'm going to spend a lot of money, I have the expectation that I am going to be serviced. I want a salesperson to come over, to talk to me, offer me coffee, show me handbags, know everything about the handbags, impress me and essentially entertain me.

In Walmart? I don't even expect the aisles to be clean let alone find a sales rep that knows anything about the handbags on display.

When you are positioning your company, you have to decide where on this spectrum you are going to be so you can build it from the start. Don't think you're going to charge $10,000 for something and provide a $50 experience. You need to map this out from the start.

Action – Decide where on the spectrum you want to position your company and decide on your ideal prices for your system.

THE POWER OF EMAIL

Day 31 – What's All The Hoopla About Emails?

Did you ever wonder what all the hoopla was about getting your email? Everywhere you look someone is trying to get you to put your email address in a box in exchange for something like a Free Report or a big promise of something exciting.

Do you know why they are doing it or what they are doing with your email address? Now I'm not about to go down dark alleys of what happens to our information, but I do want to give you a behind the scenes understanding of why an email is so valuable and why every marketer is trying so hard to get yours.

Over the next 10 days I'll give you this insight and if you own a business, I'll give you the lowdown on why you want to get in on this and how to do it.

Action – Take notice of how many times someone asks you for your email address while you are surfing on the web.

Day 32 - Why Collect Emails?

Well first and foremost it gives you a certain amount of power and freedom.

How?

Let's take my student Lori, the DNP Coach. I just recently set up her emailing campaign for her. Now whenever Lori meets someone or does any teaching whatsoever online, or goes to her website DNPCoach.com, they will see that she offers coaching on scholarly writing. Unfortunately the general in Sales is this – only about 3% of an audience is ready to buy RIGHT NOW.

We will cover more about this in a later chapter, but it means that 97% of people who find any given website either didn't know they wanted/needed your offering and/or they just aren't ready to buy for whatever reason. Therefore, a nurse might go to Lori's website and think, this is neat, but I don't need it till next year. The nurse will then bounce from Lori's website never to be seen again. Well not exactly. That nurse may remember Lori's website a year later, or Lori could spend a ton of money on advertising to stay top of mind.

Here's the thing if the user bounces and that is the end of the relationship, then that is a big loss. Not only that but it's expensive.

Now imagine instead, Lori had a way to keep in contact with that nurse, so when the nurse did need a DNP Coach, not only would she be familiar with Lori's work, but she will feel like she knows Lori better. How does this happen?

Well Lori has an opt-in on her site. If the nurse likes the opt-in and signs up for it, Lori will get that nurse's email. What she does with the email in the next step is super important.

Action – What are the last 5 opt-ins that you signed up for and why?

Day 33 – The Funnel

Yesterday we talked about why to collect emails.

This is a way how.

The way Lori's funnel works is like this: A nurse visits Lori's site DNPCoach.com. Like we said yesterday, if the nurse isn't part of the 3% of people who are ready to buy, she will bounce from the website and Lori will need to spend money over a period of time to try to get her back to her site again and again – very expensive and time consuming!

An alternative is for Lori to create a really great opt-in that the nurse would be willing to trade her email for. Now the opt-in can be anything from join my newsletter (not compelling or effective) to get a free 15 minute consultation to a coupon to whatever you want. Obviously it has to be something that your audience would want.

In Lori's case we created a template for DNP students to use when they are doing their DNP project to stay organized. Even if someone weren't ready to pay for coaching and the DNP project was a year down the line, a free template on how to structure your project is compelling for many students. It will likely occur to them that they may forget about Lori's site or how to find it when they need it, so they will sign up to make sure they grab that template for when they need it.

The beauty of the funnel is when the nurse signs up for her free report her email address goes into what we call an automation. Without Lori doing anything, the nurse will receive an automatic email thanking her for signing up for the freebie, a link to the freebie will be sent to the nurse's email inbox and Lori now has a way to market for free and stay top of mind.

Lori's funnel will take the user through an experience, where she introduces herself, gives the user some useful information on starting a DNP project or a DNP program and generally tries to connect with the reader. The initial welcome series of emails should be about 1 email every 2 days for a week, followed by an email every week or every two weeks, or even just periodically.

Think about what you could offer your audience for free that they would give you an email address for. Your opt-in should be short, easy to follow and give a quick win. You can easily create a beautiful opt-in on canva and store in a Google drive for downloading.

Sure that's neat, but then what? How does the email translate into money?

Action – What could you give your audience for free that would be useful, unique, and compelling enough to trade for their email address?

Day 34 – Show Me The Money

Ok, Lori has an opt-in and a funnel that takes a user through an email experience, but where's the money? The money comes over time in 2 different ways.

First, with Lori's continued email campaign she will remain top of mind of that user.

When and if that nurse starts a DNP project and needs help, she knows exactly who to call because she has received emails from Lori for weeks, months, maybe even years. Even if that user has never opened a single email from Lori, with repetition and frequency, she has seen her name in her inbox over and over again.

This creates a familiarity. When the user finally does need a DNP Coach or knows someone who needs a coach, Lori will be top of mind and familiar. The email funnel does not guarantee Lori will get the business, but it certainly gives her a significant advantage.

All things else equal, people would rather do business with people they know, like and trust. Familiarity is a huge benefit in marketing and the great part is, it doesn't cost Lori a penny.

The first way that Lori makes money is through repetition and frequency of her message.

The second way, is a cost savings. Ever try a Facebook campaign or look into advertising costs? Do you know how expensive those things are? The problem with advertising is that you still need to adhere to repetition and frequency in order to stay top of mind.

This is why you see the same ads over and over again. In the advertising world, 7-13 touch points are required before a person will ever consider buying from you. Unless you have a massive advertising budget, this is out of touch for small business owners.

On the other hand, do you know how much it costs to send an email? Nothing. You can send an email once a week, once a day, you could send one 5x a day and it still costs nothing more than your email service provider costs.

This is huge! While someone else can spend thousands on Facebook ads, Lori can send out automated weekly emails that keep her top of mind for free to a warm audience – that is people who have raised their hand and said, yes this is something of interest to me.

An email address is estimated to be worth about $5 per address when you look at it from direct sales and a cost savings perspective.

Tomorrow, I will tell you a little more about email marketing funnels.

Action – Start looking into Email Service Providers and compare them. For beginners, I would recommend checking out Active Campaign and Mailchimp to start. Don't buy anything yet, we'll talk more about these later, just do a little investigation.

Day 35 – The Welcome Sequence

Email marketing funnels are key. Imagine these 2 different scenarios. Let's say you set up an opt-in such as "Download my free guide". The person enters their email and gets the guide.

If that is the end of the story, then what was the point? The point of email marketing is to send emails on a regular basis marketing your business.

The second scenario is to set up the opt-in so a person enters their email address, gets the download and then is entered into a Welcome Sequence. A Welcome Sequence is a series of 3-5 emails that helps you create a relationship with your audience.

Once they know who you are, you will remain top of mind, which the entire purpose of email marketing.

Now there is an entire art and science behind email marketing campaigns, so I don't want to overwhelm at this point. What I want you to be aware of is the importance of collecting emails.

Even if you are in the worst case scenario where you capture an email and do nothing with it, it's not ideal but it's better than having no email addresses. You can always re-engage an audience at a later time.

Ok, so what do you say when you set up a Welcome Sequence? Find out tomorrow.

Action – Keep working on creating your opt-in so we can set up your first automation

Day 36 – Writing The Welcome Sequence

A Welcome Sequence is fairly self explanatory. It's a way to make your new email subscribers feel welcomed into your community. Your goal is essentially to indoctrinate your new guests into your space - kind of like into your home. You wouldn't offer someone a drink at your house and then go out shopping. So think of email in the same way.

You have offered a gift to your audience, if they accept (by way of entering their email address), then be a gracious host. I gifting you my email templates on how to write a welcome sequence. Simply go to: https://tinyurl.com/100daysWelcome to download them. Please feel free to use these emails and modify them in your own voice.

We'll keep this short so you can get moving on this task!

Action – Download your free Welcome Email Sequence and modify it for your audience - tinyurl.com/100daysWelcome

Day 37 – Email Frequency

How frequently should you email? This depends on you. You must think of your email list as a relationship. You get out of it what you put into it.

If you ignore your email list, then it will have very little value. There are a lot of big name marketing gurus who have 100k or 1 million email subscribers, but they are completely disengaged. It's a completely one sided passive relationship. This list is not effective in email marketing because if you send out an email once in a while or you are always selling people will either ignore you or unsubscribe.

If you pound your email list with ads and buy now propositions, people will get tired of you. Please remember that no one wants to be sold to, just be a valuable source in your audience's life for now.

If you provide value in your emails, you can email once a month, twice a month, once a week (recommended at a minimum), daily, twice daily… whatever you want. People who love your emails and who are interested in your business will actually read your emails.

You can even set up an automation that happens after the Welcome Sequence where your write an email once and then send all new subscribers through a Forever Sequence.

Let's say you want people to receive a minimum of 1 email a week. Well you can write 52 emails today set them up on an automation and after your audience enters your Welcome Sequence, they then continue on the Forever Sequence where they receive 1 email a week for 52+ weeks (however many emails you write).

Yes of course it's a lot of work up front, but you can tell your story over 52 weeks and really engage your audience. You build your likability factor and you don't have to write an email once a week for the rest of your life. It's one and down, but every person who comes into your funnel gets the same exact experience.

Remember branding?? This is it, the hard core stuff. Don't just throw anything together, remember if you are Gucci, you need to send Gucci-caliber emails.

What if they unsubscribe? More on that tomorrow…

Action – Decide how many emails you want your audience to receive and what their experience will be like entering into your email funnel.

Day 38 – The Unsubscriber

In email marketing we focus so much on the number of subscribers we have. It's like bragging rights or a moment of chest pounding, but the number is silly. Who cares? The mark of success isn't how many people are on your list, rather how much business you generate from your list.

What if you send an email and people start to unsubscribe? I know this is hard to believe, but for a long time I was super sensitive about this. If I sent out an email and 1 person unsubscribed after the email, I would analyze it to death. Was my email bad? Did I say something wrong? Do they not like me?

When I first started my email list, I was actually afraid of it. I was so excited to get people on my list and grow it, but then became paralyzed with fear – what if I said something that people didn't like? What if they – Unsubscribed???? Oh the humiliating failure……

I have thousands and thousands of nurses on my list, and yet a single unsubscribe would actually hurt my feelings. Talk about being sensitive! I later came to realize that it's usually not personal. Of course if you are sending out offensive emails, it might be, but there are many reasons people unsubscribe.

1. They aren't really interested in your business. So if they unsubscribe, that isn't a bad thing.
2. They don't find you interesting. This was a hard one for me to handle. But it's true. Not everyone in your potential audience is going to "jive" with you.
3. They really just wanted the download.
4. They are decluttering their inbox. I finally accepted unsubscribes when I went through my inbox and unsubscribed from every list I was on. I realized it wasn't personal, I'm just tired of all the emails.

Regardless of the reason, it's not for you to dwell on. Keep focused on finding an audience who does like to hear from you. After all a list of 1000 engaged readers is worth 100x a list with a million subscribers who don't care. You can generate a million dollar business with 1000 raving fans very easily.

Action – Decide to not worry about unsubscribes and focus all your energy on the people who actually open and engage with your emails. If you are on Active Campaign, you can monitor these metrics.

Day 39 – The Email Service Provider

Yesterday we spoke about unsubscribe, so today I want to make sure you actually have an unsubscribe button on your emails. If you are running a business and collecting emails you MUST have an email service provider.

There is no way around this. You can get a free service like MailChimp, but you must have something.

Do NOT do this. Send out a mass email from your gmail/yahoo/hotmail account. There must be a way to get off your list. If I download a brochure from you in exchange for my email, the law insists that I have the option to get off your list.

You see the unsubscribe buttons in all the ads and commercial emails you get. If you don't have an unsubscribe, people can report your emails as SPAM. You can be fined and have your email account shut down. So don't do it.

With a free option like MailChimp, there is no excuse not to set an email service provider up.

Go ahead and do that right now. If you want an inexpensive and super robust option, I would encourage you to check out Active Campaign. This is the email service provider I use. It will cost $9 a month and you will have access to an incredible customer relationship management system (CRM).

You will be able to set up automations with ease, collect data on your subscribers, follow metrics and essential run your entire business passively for $9 a month.

I strongly recommend Active Campaign over Mail Chimp for 2 reasons. If you want Mail Chimp to do automations, you need to set up their paid service which is $10/month and second there is a forced double opt-in with Mail Chimp, so when someone signs up for your download, they are forced to confirm their email addresses before you get access to it.

You will lose a ton of emails this way because people either don't confirm, or don't see that email because it ends up in their SPAM box. You can turn off the double opt-in on Active Campaign and remove the branding.

Action – Choose an email service provider (I strongly recommend Active Campaign because it's robust and full service at a very inexpensive rate) and upload your Welcome Sequence to an automation.

Day 40 – Your Email Marketing Plan

In this final email on email marketing, I want to talk about the type of emails you are going to send your audience. If you really want to be well known with your audience, the absolute key to a booming business is providing value.

At least 90% of your emails should be all value.

Please, please, please teach your audience something, give them value, make them care about you. Tell them stories, let them get to know you better. This is something that can be hard to do. And maybe it feels like you are talking to no one because most people don't respond to your emails. However, that doesn't mean they aren't effective. I can't tell you how many times I thought the whole thing was pointless and a waste of my time, then I receive an email from a subscriber who said I changed her life or she was going to pursue her dream.

Honestly, even if you help 1 person, it's worth it. But the truth is you are going to help more people than you imagine, even if they don't tell you (though I promise they will!)

Let your audience know you, the more invested they will become with you emotionally, and the more likely they will be to invest in your business when the time comes.

Now if you follow the 90% rule, if you send 4 emails a month, you can sell in one email, but make the other 3 emails completely sales free, just provide pure value. There is nothing more powerful than giving, giving and giving some more when it comes to business. And as nurses we are true experts in this area. Use your instincts and get that email list started.

Your first milestone is 500 subscribers.

Action – Create your email marketing plan, get your opt-in on your website and connect it to your email service provider. Get your first 500 subscribers.

BORING LEGALESE

Day 41 – Which Comes First?

For the next 10 days I will be writing about some legal stuff, insurance stuff and about regulations, business plans, etc.

Interestingly I find this is an area where nurses get hung up. I've heard nurses say "I can't start a business, I don't have a business plan" or "I wouldn't even know where to get started with setting up a business". The implication is they don't know the legal mambo jambo for setting up a business, but that isn't what comes first anyway.

Earlier in this book we spoke about blogging, setting up a website, how to brand yourself and email marketing. All of this can be and needs to be done PRIOR to the official unveiling of your business. You don't need to spend a dime to start your business and you shouldn't spend any money until you flesh out what it is that you are selling.

When I coach nurses through the business process I teach them to find out what they want to do with their lives, uncover their expertise and their passion. Then I teach them to find an audience in that passion and find out what their problems are. Finally, the business is to provide a solution to the problems that you found.

Then and only then do you have something to blog about, something to build a website around, something to brand and something to attract customers with.

In the beginning you should provide your services for free in exchange for testimonials and to build your credibility in your space. When you have done all that and you are ready to start your business the first thing you need is a legal structure.

Action – Make sure you are clear on what your business is prior to setting up insurances and legal structures because it will change depending on what you are offering.

Day 42 – The Legal Structure

When you start a business and make it official, you set up a legal structure around your business. This means you publicly announce you are open for business not just to your customers but also to the IRS. There are quite a few advantages to this process, so it's essential that you do this.

Now total transparency and disclaimer: I am not a lawyer nor do I pretend to be a lawyer. Your first major expense will be lawyer fees. Yes, I know it sucks. It's like buying a house and instead of making cosmetic changes you have to replace the piping.

Same idea.

But I want to lay out some options for you in terms of what is available. Now you can start a corporation, a partnership, an LLC or a sole proprietorship.

For most of you, a corporation or a partnership is going to be highly undesirable. In some circumstances it may make sense, hence get a lawyer, but in most cases it doesn't.

A standard corporation sounds nice and fancy, but it comes with a lot of requirements of how you must run the business. A corporation also gets taxed at the corporate rate. If you make $10,000 in your business, the business gets taxed at the corporate rate. Then when you pay yourself, you get taxed at the personal income level. Yes, it's so unfair, double taxation, but that's another conversation. It is what it is here and it's a killer for small businesses.

This is the main reason why a corporation as a legal structure is a bad idea for solopreneurs. Partnerships are essentially the same thing as a sole proprietorship but with multiple sole proprietors. The pro to a partnership is that you share the wealth of the company equally. The con is that you share the debts and liabilities equally.

Partnerships are typically for law firms and other types of practices like accounting or tax offices. Typically a partnership is not for start-ups.

Which leaves LLC and sole proprietorships as the mainstay of legal structure for small business.

Tomorrow, I'll talk about the pros and cons of the sole proprietorship.

Action – Find a good lawyer who is inexpensive and specializes in start-up health care businesses. Do some more research on legal structures. The fewer questions you ask the lawyer, the less expensive the visit will be.

Day 43 – Sole Proprietorship

The sole proprietorship is a small business run by a single individual. The benefit of a sole proprietorship is that it is super simple to set up, there aren't any business forms to manufacture.

You simply need to declare that you are running a business and keep your personal and business finances separate. You declare everything under your own social security number when it comes to taxes, you get some business write offs and that's it. Sounds great right? Well hold on, the downside to a sole proprietorship is the dark side. If you get sued under a sole proprietorship everything is at stake - your house, your car, your savings…

Now I don't want to scare people. There are certain industries that simply don't require anything more than a sole proprietorship. If you own a scrapbooking business or you are like my student Lori who coaches DNP students to write scholarly papers a sole proprietorship probably makes the most sense.

The lawsuit rate is negligible. Who is going to sue a DNP coach or a person who teaches crafts? Yes I'm sure there is a one in a million chance, but for that one in a million chance, your professional liability could cover you or other types of insurance (more on this later). For those of you (like me) who go into people's homes, take care of patients, physically touch them or change their wounds, a sole proprietorship is NOT an option.

Any type of home health business, recruiting agency, patient care company, or even coaching company should NOT be a sole proprietorship. Even NursePreneurs, my online program is an LLC. I can't risk my house and life savings on the off chance that someone sues me for who knows what. It happens. I've seen it happen to my entrepreneur friends. It's not pretty.

Just remember that in a low probability field where there is no physical interaction, a sole proprietorship is fine. But any other business should set up as an LLC and I'll tell you why tomorrow.

Action – Decide if your business fits into a sole proprietorship legal model.

Day 44 – Limited Liability Corporation (LLC)

An LLC is a great type of entity for small business owners. It's easy to set up, it really doesn't cost that much. I spent $250 and got my LLC set up in a matter of days.

In most cases an LLC is appropriate. Sometimes, especially if you are business partners with a physician you may need to set up a professional LLC (PLLC). Check with your state department of revenue.

Why an LLC? An LLC is a separate entity from you. It legally stands by itself. If the LLC gets sued, you are not personally liable. If the LLC has debts and you declare bankruptcy on the LLC, no bank can come after you. The caveat here is that most banks won't lend any money to an LLC without a personal guarantee, which means if the LLC does dissolve they can and will come after you for debt. Remember the bank always wins.

Now the nice thing about an LLC is that it is a pass-through entity. What does that mean? Well unlike corporations, which get taxed at the corporate rate and then you get taxed at the personal income level, an LLC does NOT get taxed.

All the money that comes through an LLC passes through straight into your pocket. You can write off business expenses to reduce the amount of money that comes into your pocket, but you are only taxed one time at the personal income tax level.

Now this is fine if your business is only pulling in $10-50,000/year. Your income bracket won't go up that much. When your business starts bringing in $1,000,000 a year, you may need to re-evaluate your legal structure.

The pros are a lower tax rate, reduced exposure to legal issues and it's simple to put together.

The cons are the set-up fee, keeping minutes and having completely separate records for everything including a separate bank account, credit cards, etc.

Finally a word to the wise. Set your business up in the state where you live. One of my first businesses I set up I did in the state of Delaware for the "tax advantages". Only to find out that the tax advantages were for real corporations and not small business owners. Not only did I have to pay taxes in Delaware but in Pennsylvania as well. When I shut down my Delaware LLC it cost me $500. It was incredibly painful and expensive.

There are no tax advantages for start-ups really in other states. Just set up the process in your home state. When money starts rolling and you are paying horrendous tax bills then maybe it will be worth it. My biggest wish for you is that you have this problem and you have to start paying out the big bucks for lawyers to restructure your legal status.

Action – Decide if the LLC is for you. If your business is ready to go, choose a company to set up your legal structure or go to your state's department of revenue and do it yourself.

Day 45 – The Business Plan

You have your legal structure in place. Now what? Many nurses get hung up on a business plan. I had this conversation recently with my sister. I told her she should start a business selling pet parties to rich people. She thought it was a good idea at the time, but then when I asked her later she said "It's not going to happen I don't even have a business plan". I was like what???

Who cares? You don't need a traditional academic business plan. I did an MBA, I had to write business plans all the time.

At the time I thought they were stupid and useless and I still think they are. Most major Ivy leagues MBA programs agree with me and they have done away with them.

The traditional business plan for start-ups does not make any sense at all. Try projecting out 5 years on something you have no idea of what it's going to look like in 5 weeks.

The only time a business plan is needed is if you are asking the bank or angel investors for money. Otherwise a business plan is a waste of time. If you need large sums of money to start your business, this is the wrong book for you sorry to say! I help nurses start up a business from within based on their knowledge and expertise, I don't bring medical devices to market.

If you want to start a clinic, home health agency or staffing firm you will need a ton of money. These types of businesses are very risky, very different and you need a very different mentor!

Does that mean your business is a free for all with no planning required? Of course not. What you need is something more in line with a vision board. Tomorrow I will give you that vision board so you can see where your business is going.

Action – Scrap the idea of a traditional business plan.

Day 46 – The Lean Machine

One of the reasons I say that obtaining an MBA is not only a waste of time if you want to start a business, it actually puts you 2 steps backwards. An MBA is great if you want to climb the corporate ladder, and it's a necessity. If you actually want to start a business, the MBA will teach you the wrong things to do.

One of the first myths that MBAs perpetuate is the need for a business plan. A formal business plan doesn't make any sense at all for a solopreneur. If a business plan doesn't serve you and you aren't borrowing money than it simply becomes an academic exercise.

What many flexible business programs with an entrepreneurial focus are doing is getting rid of the business plan in favor of the Lean Canvas. In doctoral nursing programs we are doing this as well. The Lean Canvas allows you to map out your idea and provide you with a vision of where you are going.

You can download a copy of the Lean Canvas that I teach in my program NursePreneurs by following this link: tinyurl.com/leannurses. It's much easier to look at, much easier to complete and more useful than a formal business plan.

Remember companies like Walmart, Google, Facebook and Nike never had a business plan (because they aren't useful in the beginning). By the time they got to be major corporations, yes of course they integrated business plans, but not for the first several years.

How can you project 5 years out and amortize equipment and properties you don't have? This is just silly. When you are starting a business, focus on your Vision, Mission and Values, know what your solution is and deliver it. As the money starts flowing in and you want to hire MBAs to do your business plan that is great. Until then, if you aren't borrowing money from the bank, use the Lean Canvas to guide your first year.

Action – Download the Lean Canvas template and create your first "business plan". Go to tinyurl.com/leannurses

Day 47 – Professional Liability Insurance

One way that you absolutely must protect yourself in your start-up business is to purchase professional liability insurance.

As a nurse, even if you aren't doing "nursing" things, you are held to that standard. Please do not start a business without buying professional liability insurance. You must have it. It's not very expensive especially for nurses. Because nurses aren't sued on a regular basis, insurance is super cheap, like less than $100 a year.

Look to companies like NSO or CM&F. The most expensive insurance I had was a yearly rate of $1500. This covered me in the operating room as a first assist as well as for injecting cosmetic fillers and botox. If you aren't doing those things your insurance will be much less.

Now if you are a midwife or do anything with pregnant women or with anesthesia this rate will be much, much higher.

I'm keeping this short because I want you to act. Even if you don't start a business, getting professional liability insurance is not a waste of money. Do this first and do it now.

Action – Go purchase professional liability insurance.

Day 48 – Insurance Policies

Now there are lots of types of insurance policies out there, what do you really need?

There are:

- General liability insurance
- Worker's compensation
- Property insurance
- Commercial property insurance
- Product liability insurance
- Vehicle insurance
- Business interruption insurance.

Do you really need all this insurance? Well it depends on the type of business you own. Let's look at the different types, and then you can decide what is right for you. Not everyone needs all of these. Insurance is picking and choosing what is right for you and your business.

General Liability

General liability insurance protects your company's assets and will pay for obligations such as medical costs if someone gets hurt on your property. If you are a home based business but have people come to your house, this may be something you need.

General liability can also cover your legal defense if you are sued. It can cover claims of false or misleading advertising, libel, slander and copyright infringement.

Worker's Compensation

If you don't have employees you clearly don't need worker's compensation. When you do have employees, this will be something you need to look into.

Property Insurance

If you are renting a space or you own it, you must have property insurance. This will cover equipment, signage, inventory and furniture in the event of fire, storm or theft.

Commercial Property Insurance

If you are a home based business, you may want to look into adding commercial property insurance to your homeowners policy. Homeowners will generally not cover damage to business property in your home.

Product Liability Insurance

If your business manufactures products for sale on the general market, product liability insurance is a must. Even a business that takes every measure possible to make sure its products are safe can find itself named in a lawsuit due to damages caused by one of its products.

Vehicle Insurance

If company vehicles will be used, those vehicles should be fully insured to protect businesses against liability if an accident should occur. This will likely not be needed in a 1 person start up show!

Business Interruption Insurance

If your business becomes your full time job and an interruption in service would cause you significant hardship, then business interruption insurance is necessary, otherwise don't worry about this for now. This type of insurance is especially applicable to companies that require a physical location to do business, such as retail stores.

By having the right insurance in place, a business can avoid a major financial loss due to a lawsuit or catastrophic event. Check with your insurer to find out what forms of insurance are advised for your type of business and put those plans in place as soon as possible.

Action – Call a few insurance companies and ask them their opinion on what you need. Get at least 3 different opinions and quotes.

Day 49 – Bonded & Insured

Ever see websites where they say we are licensed, bonded and insured? Well you are a licensed nurse, you hopefully got professional insurance a couple days ago, now the question is, do you need to be bonded as well and what does that mean?

Bonds are meant to protect consumers. If you work in a business that conducts business in a client's home, you might want to consider getting bonded. The first purpose of a bond is to reassure the customers. The assurance is that the business will be conducted in accordance with the law—and if it isn't, the bond will provide protection.

Bonds protect the client from theft or damage to their property. For instance if you are a cleaning company, you would get bonded in case your cleaners broke property or stole property from a house.

If you are working solo, you might consider getting a bond, not for you but for the reassurance to the client that you are professional and reliable.

Action – Call a couple bonding agencies to see if your company would even qualify. Get at least 3 quotes before you consider signing anything.

Day 50 - Regulations

What kind of regulations do you need to adhere to when you start a business? This will vary tremendously. For instance there is a very fine line between "concierge nursing" and "home care".

Home care is tightly regulated by different governing bodies. There are lots of rules and regulations that you must adhere to. Don't try to wing it. There are agencies whose sole purpose is to shut people down or discover Medicare/Medicaid fraud. Saying you "didn't know" won't hold water. You will know and you will get financially penalized with potential prison time!

If you start a home care business, clinic, or staffing agency, you MUST know the regulations → the present and the ones that are coming.

Concierge nursing is not regulated. Mallory Buxton, who runs Solos Nurse, a concierge nurse business is an ICU nurse who started her business. She does not have a medical director, she does not follow Medicare rules and she gets paid a ton of money to provide what nursing do best - care and teaching her expertise.

IV hydration is another business that is highly unregulated. What do you need to set up? Well, Christie from CityHydration.com is an associate degree nurse who pays a medical director to write her standing orders for her. She also paid a pharmacist to help her formulate her bags, which the physician orders.

→Aside from that there is no regulation.
→Want to be a nurse coach - no regulations.
→ Want to be a consultant - no regulations.

Before you start any business make sure you consult a lawyer to help you know when you've crossed line that puts your nursing license at risk. And make sure you buy professional liability insurance!

Action – Call your lawyer!

GET CLIENTS NOW

Day 51 – Sell By Not Selling

When I put together this topic of ways to get clients in your business, I quickly became overwhelmed. There are so many things you could do, how am I going to address all this in 10 days?

Well, I can't clearly. But I do want to touch on some elements of what you really need to focus on.

To kick this section about getting clients off, I want to start with a reminder to everyone that business is about relationships.

Getting clients is about creating a network of meaningful relationships. As nurses we are great at doing that. As business owners, not so much.

People love to buy, but hate being sold to.

If you can appreciate and internalize this statement then everything I say from here on out will resonate with you.

For example, in my Facebook Group: Business + Marketing for NursePreneurs, I have a no soliciting policy. Is it because I don't want nurses to make money or steal nurses away?

No.

It's because it's annoying to have a bunch of people hacking their stuff without contributing anything.

Be mindful and respectful of others. By contributing information others will come to see you as valuable and want to work with you. Just because you are online and not in someone's house doesn't mean all etiquette gets brushed aside.

Here is another example of a nurse who starts selling her stuff in the middle of a work text email.

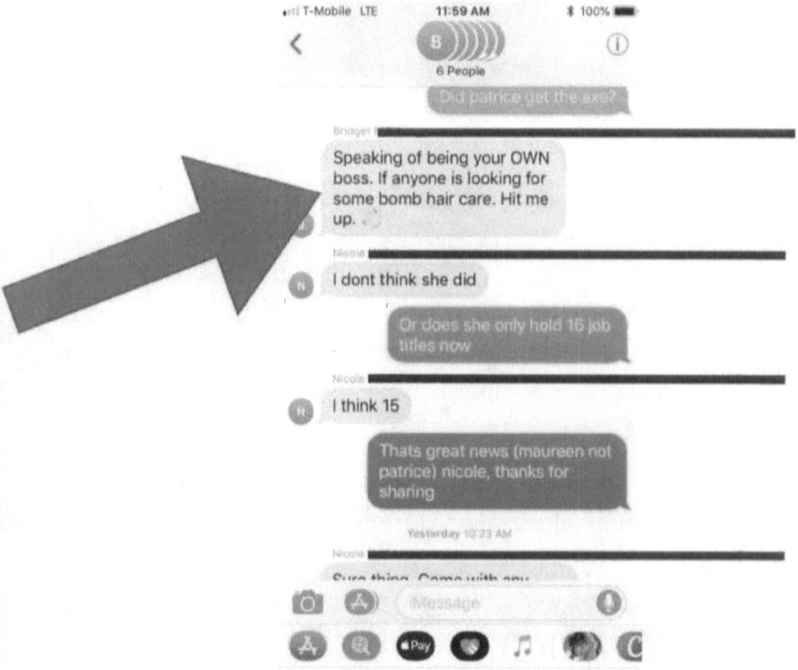

Really?

In case no one else is telling you, I am - it's soooo annoying when someone is constantly selling…. They don't get sales, they just irritate people and make them run them away, they destroy Facebook groups, they turn LinkedIn groups into recruitment campaigns. Most importantly, they destroy relationships. What I'm telling you is that business is all about relationships. Don't destroy them, build them up.

In this section I want to show **what you should be doing** as a respectable and intelligent business owner. If you're not yet a business owner, you can still use this template as a marketing plan for when you do have a business.

Action – If you are "selling" to friends and family – STOP immediately. Just be a friend, give advice, teach what you know and you will reap the benefits. This is also how you become an excellent business owner.

Day 52 – What Do You Do?

How you answer the question of "what do you do" is a make or break event that you must master. Don't throw away this opportunity. It's the one opportunity you have to pitch your business, without being sleazy or coming off pushy.

Someone is literally allowing you to pitch them, so be prepared for it.

If you answer:
"Oh I'm just a nurse"

What kind of predicament do you put your listener in? You'll get some kind of response like, "oh my mother was a nurse. Yeah she loved it, it's great, well I'm going to get another drink". Or the person will say “oh that’s nice, do you like it?” Either way, the conversation doesn’t go the way it could. You can make the answer to this question very exciting.

Let's go over some messages you might pre-prepare. Now, you want to focus on outcomes of what you offer and integrate that into your response. Then you practice your response until it becomes your unconscious competence.

That means if you have to say your statement 100 x to remember it, then do it. It's the most worthwhile thing you will do for your own business.

Try coming up with a response such as I help (your audience) to (what benefit do they want to achieve).

Examples:

If you are a Rodan + Fields consultant, this is the time to tell the listener:
"I help women look ageless, timeless and confident"

If you are a coach maybe you say:
"I help people with diabetes come off their medications within 90 days."

My student Lori who teaches scholarly writing could say:

"I prepare DNP students to ace their dissertation project review and publish their capstone projects within 90 days of graduation".

You want someone to physically turn towards you and say:
"Really, how do you do that?"

This is when you can go into an example of a problem, then provide your solution. You are pitching but the person you are talking to doesn't realize it. Their guard is down and they are open to hearing what you have to say. The other great part of this is that they feel like they've "discovered" you. They were lucky enough to have met you. This is powerful!

Think about the amazing outcomes you bring to people.

Action – Answer the question what do you do? Use the framework of this sentence: I help (audience) to (achieve what benefit/outcome).

Day 53 – The Dream 100

The Dream 100 is a potent method for getting clients. If you focus on just this one technique you will get more sales.

Here's how it works. Find 100 people/clients/businesses that are your perfect match for your business.

For instance, in my Concierge Nurse Services business, I found a list of 100 plastic surgeons I wanted to work with. With NursePreneurs, I made a list of the top 100 nurses who were most interactive with my emails and on my site and with Hydration Operation, I made a list of 100 businesses who I thought would make great partners.

Why?

Because it's much easier to deal with 100 people than tens of thousands of people. If you can prove your process and your business, get testimonials and referrals from 100 people, you will have a thriving business.

Start with 100 people because it's manageable and accessible. You can really focus on getting to know them. Connect on social media, participate in their conversations, like their Instagram pictures, give useful advice, etc.

For individuals, I connect with them on social media, send them private messages and emails that provide value to them. If you don't provide some kind of value, then you will be harassing them, so keep that in mind. When I'm working business to business I send letters, emails and helpful information ON A CONSISTENT basis. Not once, not twice, but every other week.

Your perfect client may not be ready to buy today. In fact only 3% of any given audience is ready to buy exactly what you are selling today. If you only focus on 3%, you are missing out on the 97% that could be part of your business tomorrow or the next day, or even 2 years from today.

You need to build a relationship with people and social media has made it so easy.

You see if you make 1 comment or send 1 email, this is ineffective. You have to be persistent. Think about that real estate agent who faithfully sends listings in your area every month without fail. You probably aren't listing your house for sale today, tomorrow or next month. However, if 1 year from now you do, that real estate agent is going to be top of mind. Or if a friend of yours is listing, you can give that person's name and contact information.

Business is about relationships and referrals. Spend your time on these two things and you will be successful. Start with your Dream 100 so it's not overwhelming. You can manage 100 new contacts.

Action – Create a list of 100 people who you want to connect with and then connect with them via social media or other method.

Day 54 – The 7 Musts Of Marketing

Chet Holmes talks about the 7 Musts of Marketing, and if you haven't read his book The Ultimate_Sales_Machine, you are missing out!

This is hands down the most useful marketing guide I've ever used. I'm going to talk about each one of his ideas over the course of the next 7 days, but I can in no way do it justice. Buy that book and refer to it often.

The first Must of Marketing according Chet is Internet Presence. Earlier in this book we talked about which type of website to set up, but there is more to it then just your homepage.

For instance, if you hear about a new product or service, what is the first thing you do? You Google it of course. Well when people hear about you, they will Google you as well. What will people find when they Google your name or business?

Do you even come up?

Here is a statistic to remember. If someone is actively searching to buy something they will rarely make it past page 1 of any Google search. **Close to 99% of people find what they are looking for on page 1 of a Google search.** Think about that for a second...

Now if they are looking for what your business does, how are they going to find you? Unless someone goes to your exact website (and can actually spell it correctly), how else do they find you?

This is SEO - search engine optimization. You don't have to hire an expensive SEO manager, but you do need to put out content on the web to be found.

Blogging particularly on specific keywords is extremely helpful, but if no one is coming to your blog, it likely won't reach a critical mass. Consider guest blogging on other sites who actually have traffic. For instance if I write an article on my own blog, it gets a trickle of traffic. If I post on AllNurses.com or Nurse.com, OMG - there are millions of potential views.

Guest blogging on popular websites is a great way to get your name out there.

Also make sure you optimize your LinkedIn account to say what you want to be known for. When I was searching for nurse authors who specialized in a particular field like Endocrine or Nephrology, I found who I was looking for on LinkedIn.

LinkedIn has massive SEO, so make sure you use it to your advantage.

Make yourself be found by creating a presence for yourself on the Internet. Go ahead and search yourself and see how much work you need to do.

Action – Optimize your LinkedIn account for business and Google yourself and your website to see what is out there.

Day 55 – Corporate Literature

I teach my students to put a system together BEFORE they start branding themselves. It's hard to brand when you aren't clear about what you are doing. The colors, fonts, packaging, positioning, pricing - all that has to come together and not piecemeal.

Once you have the fonts and colors, you can start to make pretty brochures, business cards and corporate literature. Corporate literature is the second Musts of Marketing.

But wait..

Here's the thing. I don't want you to make brochures and flyers about you and your company. Do you know what happens to brochures and flyers about you? They get thrown away. I know this is hard to understand, but your audience isn't interested in your business or what you are selling.

They are simply interested in how you can help them. Therefore you want to make your brochures, flyers and business cards with that idea in mind. When I sent out my first postcard for Concierge Nurse Services, it was to introduce myself. Likely that postcard got thrown away after they noticed how pretty it was.

The second card I sent out was how to make a Strawberry Ginger Zinger Smoothie and Lose Weight. Now why in the world would that be an effective postcard to send out and how was that helpful to my business?

Well the card wasn't for the surgeons, it was for the patients. How many plastic surgery patients do you think would be interested in making a yummy smoothie and lose weight at the same time?

Exactly – a lot. And it's something they would keep.

My website is at the bottom with More Recipes that they can download. The card is for my business, but has nothing to do with me. Notice I didn't say "buy my stuff, download my stuff, get my stuff".

Provide value with your brochures, business cards and flyers and the business will follow.

Action – Use canva.com to design a brochure for your business. Make the brochure something that provides incredible value to your audience that would make them keep it.

Day 56 – Direct Mail

I used to think direct mail was a huge waste of time. Yet ironically I joined a mastermind group with none other than John Carlton, who is one the greatest copywriters and direct mail masters alive.

When I explained my business model to him, he told me to send direct mail.

Direct mail? You mean like the mail I throw away every day?

It seems like such a huge waste of money. Not to mention, my audience is 4 million nurses. There is no way I could ever mail a postcard to all those people.

Even the state directories have tens of thousands of nurses listed inside of them. Ugghhh, right?

Well, I never did do a direct mail campaign to nurses, only because I couldn't wrap my mind around how to do it, but when it came to Concierge Nurse Services, the value of a direct mail campaign was clearly obvious.

One of things I teach my students is the Dream 100 method for engaging their audience. You don't have to engage millions of people, you only need to engage 100 people.

With Concierge Nurse Services, I only need to engage 100 surgeon offices. It's quite easy and straightforward (and affordable) for me to send a direct mail campaign. I just told you that I sent my brochure on how to make a Strawberry Ginger Zinger Smoothie and lose weight. That was part of my direct mail campaign.

But it doesn't stop there. Oh no, this is a direct mail campaign. You don't send 1 piece of mail and call it a day.

I have mailings that go out like clockwork every other Monday. I send a newsletter (that is interesting to plastic surgeons and their staff, not about what I'm doing), I send tips, tricks and resources for their patients. I send small gifts like pen lights or pedometers - super cheap.

Please don't send anything expensive, it will come off as a bribe!

Use your brochure making skills and marketing know how to create a system for audience. Send them letters on a regular basis through first class mail. If you have a relatively small list like I do, write everything in handwriting. No need to type. It will feel much more personal and will likely get opened.

And lastly, be persistent. Have a 2-year plan. Send a piece of mail every other week for the next 2 years to your top 50-100-1000 clients and I can virtually guarantee you, you will get clients coming in.

Action – Create a direct mail campaign for the next 6 months using your Dream 100 list.

Day 57 - Personal Contact.

Personal contact is actually the most potent form of marketing you can do. You are armed with your message that you tweaked, you are having conversations with people, you are delivering value AND you never once mentioned that you had something to sell. Yet people want to know how they can work with you.

This is the power of personal contact. I already told you about my brochures and the direct mail campaign, and they were great. Except they didn't bring in the leads -- until we made personal contact.

It wasn't until I started calling the offices to follow up that I was able to secure an office to work with my company.

I notice this now with other sales reps. I recently started looking into getting an au pair to live with me and my son. There was one company that persistent in calling me every other day for weeks.

I was finally ready to secure an au pair and guess who called? And guess who won my business?

Making personal contact cannot be overstated. You can't just sit behind your computer and send out emails. You need to go where your audience is, hang out with them, provide them value. Get yourself involved in the community - it's all synergistic. It helps you, it helps them.

Action – Decide on a plan to establish more personal contact in marketing your business.

Day 58 – Market Education.

One of the most significant ways to provide value is simply to provide education. This is the clearest difference between marketing and selling.

Let me give you some examples of how you can market yourself without selling through market education:

1. Participate on groups online and offer real and valuable advice with no strings attached

2. Write an article in a journal that your audience reads

3. Create brochures that provide useful information and NOT a sales pitch

4. Speak at tradeshows or any local, national, international event

5. Hold an online summit

6. Host a webinar or series of webinars for free that teach something valuable

The key here is to teach something that the person will walk away with and think "Wow that was amazing and useful information."

Don't tease your audience. There is nothing worse than someone setting up the problem and then at the end says "Well if you want the answer, buy my stuff". This is just a sh*tty way to do business. Don't do it.

You're not going to give away too much information. What you are going to do is amass a tribe of loyal followers.

Not everyone will buy from you. Your goal isn't to sell to everyone, it's to sell to the right people at the right time.

Use market education to position yourself as an authority figure in your space.

Here is a challenge for you: Over the next month, find an online group on Facebook or LinkedIn or Quora, wherever and provide only value 3x per week. No selling, no sales pitch. Just find conversations that center around what you do and provide solutions to the group. See what happens.

I bet you will find more people will be interested in you than you can imagine.

Action – Participate on an online group 3x per week and provide value.

Day 59 – Advertising

Now when you first start out advertising may not be in the budget, but it's definitely a powerful way to establish your business. Your audience will likely not buy from you cold, at least very few do.

I've said before only 3% of any audience is ready to buy when they see your advertisement, so the key to advertising is frequency and repetition. This gets very expensive very quickly.

Facebook ads and Google ads are a good idea as well, but the cost per clicks has risen dramatically because of such fierce competition.

For example if you want to drive people to your webinar, your cost per click on Facebook might be $8 per click. That means you will need to spend $800 to get 100 people just to click on your link. With a 15% show up rate, that means you could expect 15 people to show up. With a 1% conversion rate means that maybe 1 person if anyone will buy. This is the reality of online sales.

Facebook and Google are no longer slam dunk methods of advertising. If you do choose these methods, I would strongly recommend you research them, read up as much as possible, and start low, like $5/day just to test it out.

Other ways to advertise are to buy space in trade magazines or billboards, remnant TV space, look into radio and inserts in newspapers and local magazines. Also consider your neighborhood newsletter which will be significantly cheaper.

Make sure you set up an advertising strategy that focuses on frequency and repetition. Do not waste your money to buy 1 ad. You need to buy a series of ads. Don't change your ad so it looks completely different each time. This is not a time to get creative, be consistent. Otherwise you lose the effect of repetition.

My best advice… Get started with the other Musts of Marketing first, get some money coming in and then use it to create an advertising budget. Don't start with this one.

In the next email, I'll tell you how to get FREE advertising...

Action – Decide if you have an advertising budget and how to maximize it for frequency and repetition.

Day 60 – Media

How to get free advertising? Well what could be better than media attention? Imagine you are sitting on The Today Show explaining how you help diabetic patients eat better or you are with Dr. Oz explaining the importance of sleep.

Far-fetched? Out of your reach?

No way!

It's just a matter of knowing who to contact and what to say.

I want you to remember this - 80% of media is placed (not earned). What does that mean? It means that media outlets aren't running around looking for stories, people bring their stories to them. And then the media outlets choose what resonates with them and their audience.

So if you never bring your story to the media, don't expect the media to come knocking on your door for an interview. Don't think you don't have enough experience, enough knowledge or enough experience.

One of the fastest and easiest ways to get media attention is by being available for expert opinion. How do you do that? Well sign up for free on HARO - help a reporter out. This is a site that journalist use when they need opinions from experts.

A lot of it won't be relevant, but some of it will. If a journalist uses your pitch idea as fodder for their article, you can use that article to show off your credibility and authority.

Another way is to guest post on other people's blogs, or pitch podcasters so that you can tell your story.

Finally, when all else fails, start a YouTube channel.

Don't tell me no one has ever gotten famous from a YouTube channel – Remember Justin Bieber, of course you do!

Not only is a great way to get your message out, you also show media outlets what it would be like to have you on their TV show. It's free and there is no barrier to entry except for your mindset.

We will go over video later in this book, so the seed is planted...

Action – Make a media strategy plan. Choose 10 media outlets to pitch your business idea to and then send them your pitch.

VIDEO MARKETING

Day 61 – Video Marketing

When I first thought of doing video, I literally started having a panic attack. After all how can you do video when you hate how you look on camera and you hate how you sound? Other people could do video, but not me. I was weird and awkward on camera. There was no way, no how I would ever do video.

Except, video works. It's effective. For a shy, introverted person like myself, I could practice, practice, practice in the private of my own home or office. It would mean I wouldn't have to go to networking events! (Actually that's not true you still have to go to networking events, but it was one way I convinced myself to do video).

Alas, I was petrified whenever the video button would turn red. I have some horrific video footage of myself. I mean it's bad. It's like I was trying as hard as possible to make the worst video ever. My voice was deep, soft, barely audible. My hair was in shambles, I had a sweatshirt on that was 5 sizes too big, no make-up. Really what was I thinking?

No one ever wants to see that. It was my way of proving to myself that I couldn't do it. I had to step back from that traumatic experience and say ok, how could this have been better. This was easy, because it couldn't be any worse. I thought, let me at least pull my hair back and put on a little make-up. Better. Ok, now let me wear clothes that make me feel good. Even better. Finally, let me practice projecting my voice and making eye contact with the camera. Perfect!

Well not perfect, but done is better than perfect. It was good enough.

What about you? What are your thoughts on video marketing and what would it take to get you to do a video for your business or your personal brand?

Action – Take a video of yourself and in less than 2 minutes explain what you were hoping for when you got this book? What were your expectations. Try it and save it to compare to future videos.

Day 62 – Myth #1 You Need Expensive Video Equipment

In the beginning of my business because I hated video so much, I started out with voice over Powerpoints. There were fine and a nice segue into video but I quickly realized that I needed to be the face of my business. You do too. It's the second most effective way of communicating with people (personal contact is the first and it's in a league of it's own).

In the early days of my business I decided I couldn't do video because I didn't have any video equipment, I didn't have a studio, I didn't have video editing equipment. But guess what, none of that is important. You can't use that as an excuse not to start video.

Some of the biggest names in the marketing and influencer industry use their smart phone to record themselves in a single take. Yes the very same phone you have can be your ticket to Hollywood, or at least to building your business.

The trend these days is to be real and authentic. What is more real than unpolished video of you giving tips or resources to your audience or explaining a concept?

Honestly it's so much easier to record on your smart phone too. Some of your fears of video may just be these practicalities, though I suspect, it's mostly a psychological barrier.

The good news is you don't need video equipment, you just need a smart phone. The bad news you don't need video equipment to get started, you just need a smart phone.

Now here's the big question: What do you say when the record button goes on? Ahhhh…

Action – Use your smart phone to record a second video of yourself saying your name, your hometown, your favorite food and 1 interesting thing about yourself.

Day 63 – The POSER Solution

One of the biggest fears about going on camera is having nothing to say. It's funny because we talk all day about anything and everything, yet someone turns on a camera and we become mute.

Well the best way around this is to map out some thoughts, concepts, tips and resources you want to share with your audience. What is the 1 thing you want your audience to walk away knowing?

There is a simple formula that you can follow that will work in basically any situation and will help you keep your thoughts organized. Kevin Rogers, the comedian turned A-list copywriter gave me this formula to help with video marketing. It's called the POSER formula. It's super easy and once you get the flow going, you'll be able to do this without thinking.

POSER stands for Promise, Obstacle, Solution, Example, Reach

When you start a video, start by stating the promise of your video. What do you promise your audience to talk about in your video? This has to come first. You can't expect someone to spend 5 minutes listening to your video to find out it wasn't for them. You have to tell them in the first 3 seconds if your video is worth watching or not.

Then you can talk about the obstacles of attaining whatever the promise is. Provide a couple of obstacles or just one, it's up to you. Give the solution to overcoming the obstacle. Don't tease the solution, people will get annoyed with you and stop watching your videos.

Provide an example. Don't forget this! The example is typically what people will remember, especially if it is someone that you have helped. Finally get your audience to reach out with a call to action. Don't make any video without a call to action, whether it's comment below, share with a friend, follow me on social media, etc. Always ask your audience to do something.

Example POSER Formula:

Intro (Promise) – I'm going to show you how to fly for free to the Bahamas

Obstacle – Many frequent flyer plans suck and you can never book the day you want

Solution – Use credit card points or some other solution

Example – I taught this to my friend Sue, who spent 2 weeks basking in the sun for FREE (I would show a picture of Sue in Bahamas having fun)

Reach – Share this video with someone you know who is in desperate need of a vacation

Now that's not so hard is it? Now it's your turn to give it a try.

Action – Record a video using the POSER formula on any frequently asked question people bring to you.

Day 64 – Tips For Video

Now that you have a formula, you need to make a list of topics that you want to talk about. These videos don't have to be long. The POSER formula I gave you could be a 30 second video or a 5 minute video.

When you are starting out I would recommend keeping them short. As you become more comfortable and your audience wants more then you will just know the right length. Maybe it's an hour, I don't know. It depends on you, your topic and your audience.

Something to remember is that a 30-second video may take you hours to complete when you first start out, but soon it will really only take 30 seconds. Using the POSER formula will help you to tell a story without concentrating really hard.

Next, what you want to do is to relax on the camera. The best way to relax is to set up your phone and start recording. Then, I want you tell your POSER story 15 times non-stop on camera. Don't stop the camera. Just do the first take. If you mess up, start over, but don't stop the camera.

I can tell you right now the first 5 takes are going to be horrendous and that's ok. You can delete them later. Around the 10th time you've told the same story, your mind is getting bored, your body is relaxing and you know the story by heart. The last 5 times, I want you to try to add energy, enthusiasm and change the intonation of your voice. You'll be amazed at how much better the last video is from the first.

Action – **Take your POSER formula and record the same story 10 times.**

Day 65 - Myth #2 You Need A Video Studio

Nope. And in fact I would encourage you to shoot your videos in a setting where you are most comfortable. That might be at home, on the beach, shopping in a store or wherever. Just make sure the noise around you isn't louder than your voice. Wherever you are inspired, you should make a video.

Imagine going into your local coffee shop and you think of something. Use the POSER formula and shoot the video right then and there. Too self-conscious? Write down your idea and do it later. The more you do video, the less self-conscious you will become. One day you will find yourself getting on an airplane and recording a quick 30-second video while your seatmate is wondering what kind of celebrity you are.

Look, most people are afraid of video. There is no need to be. You simply have to stretch your comfort zone to a point where you set the bar of uncomfortableness to another level. I got over my fear of video. My new fear is LIVE video and TV. I'm working on it. After I'm comfortable with LIVE video and TV, public speaking at large events? It's hard to say, but I'm going to keep on pushing.

Why are we doing video again aside from torturing a few souls?

It's important to create short videos for your audience so they can connect with you. People are more likely to do business with people they know, like and trust when all things are equal.

So if you have videos, people will feel like they know you. It will set you apart from your competition who is hiding behind advertisements and Powerpoint presentations.

Action – Make a POSER video in public, i.e. somewhere where other people can see you do it.

Day 66 - Lighting

Get your lighting right. One pro tip for video, make sure you always have the light in front of you. Regardless of what camera you are using, the lens will focus in on the light. If you are sitting in front of a window, you will appear dark, this is no good. You want light coming into the room. Instead of sitting in front of the window put the camera in front of the window. This way, the light will come in but you won't be washed out.

Remember this particularly when you are out and about. Beware of windows behind you. You want to capture the light, but not in the frame of the video.

If you are in a room without lights, you can use 2 separate lights placed at 45 degrees in front of you on your right and left. Any light will do. You don't need to buy expensive studio lights, just a regular lamp will do.

Now this is an example of how light can wash you out...

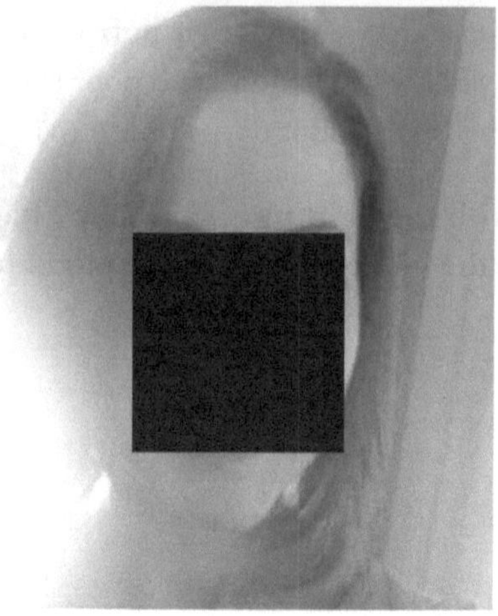

And this is an example of how light can make you dark and creepy. The light must always be in front of you. Beware of any window in your video.

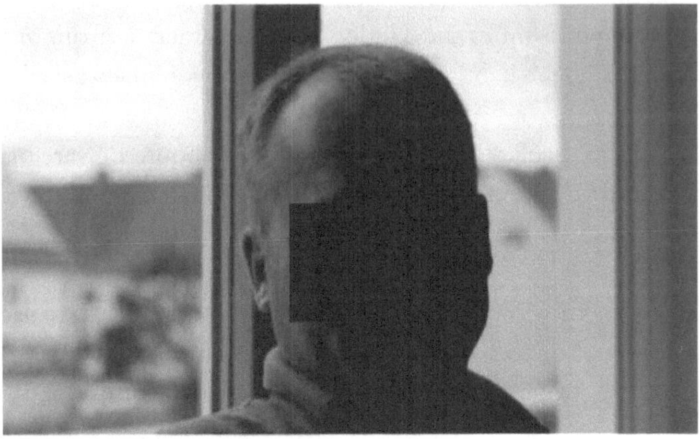

Keeping two lights at a 45 degree angle in front of you can make all the difference. You will create shadows and poor skin texture if your angles are off. Good lighting is key and it doesn't need to be fancy.

Action – Play with the lighting. Take some bad pictures and fix them with the tips in the video so you understand how to play with light.

Day 67 – Myth #3 You Need Professional Editing Equipment

This is totally bogus. You do not need expensive video editing equipment. If you want you can use imovie or whatever free program comes with your computer. I would highly recommend, though that you check out this blog post I did on Movavi (tinyurl.com/NurseMovavi). You can get Movavi pretty cheaply, especially using the trick I teach you in this post.

Movavi is highly intuitive and very easy to learn. In no time you will be sending out pretty crafty video edits with lots of animation, text and backdrops. Or you can do what a lot of influencers do, keep it raw and shoot in 1 take (or a couple takes), and send your video right to social media from your phone. No editing required. This of course does not mean no practicing required. You must practice to get comfortable on video.

Action – Check out the Movavi post and then Movavi software. Decide if you are ready to invest in this software

Day 68 – Sound

Sound is important, but you will find that the sound quality on your phone or computer is sufficient. Does a microphone sound better?

Yes of course it does. Is it worth the hassle and money to buy a microphone?

Not right away.

First things first.

Start taking videos.
Unless there is so much background noise that no one can hear you, then very few people would ever complain about your audio not being "professional grade". In fact, it goes back to the feeling of authenticity that you get when you use just what you have available to you.

If you want to practice with sound, download the free software called Audacity. You will learn a ton about sound, how you sound, how the audio on your computer sounds, how it differs from a microphone sound. You can also record podcasts, phone interviews, etc on Audacity. It's a terrific program.

Action – Check out Audacity and download it for free. Then look at the cost of microphones. If you are gung-ho to do video then invest in the $50 range with a USB connection to start. You can upgrade later.

Day 69 – Video Slick

Video-slick and polished is now becoming old school. In fact, most mainstream influencers do not invest in or use high tech video equipment.

The good news is that you don't need to spend money to do video!

The bad news is that you have no excuse NOT to do video.

The only way to truly get good at this is to practice, practice, practice. In fact, I have a challenge for you today to help you with getting good on video.

What I want you to do is to make a list of 10 common objections your audience would have to investing in your business or a business that you are thinking of starting. I want you to come up with a response to these objections in 2 minutes or less and record yourself.

This exercise has several layers to it, so don't think it's a waste of time.

1. It forces you to think about what people will object to in your business
2. It will make you reflect on how your product, service or idea can overcome this objection
3. If you can't overcome the objection, think about what you could do to overcome the objection
4. Find the words to overcome the objection quickly
5. And of course, practice your video skills.

When you are done, watch the videos. Evaluate the quality of the sound, lighting and environment. Also while you are at evaluate how believable you are at overcoming objections! If you take an hour out of your day to do this, or maybe record one objection a day for 10 days, I promise you by the end of it, you will have a solid FAQs for your business AND you will find a new comfort level with video.

Action – Record the answer to 10 FAQs that people routinely ask you.

Day 70 – Download My Free Book

For my final action on the video marketing segment, I would love to gift you the book I wrote for Video Marketing, yours completely FREE! Enjoy!

Action – Go to: tinyurl.com/NurseVideoMarketing to claim your book.

WEBINARS THAT SELL

Day 71 – Webinars?

Why webinars? How does this fit into the 100 Days of Action to build an online nursing business? Well, webinars are a great way to get noticed, they are jammed pack with information and you effectively can sell yourself through your knowledge and leadership. After all, running a business makes you a leader. Your ultimate goal is to help people to go where they want.

As you move forward or even think about moving forward in the process of starting a business, keep webinars in your mind. You can post them on social media, you can share them, you can invite people to attend. You can even hold virtual summits and invite influencers to be part of your process.

It's a huge credibility booster having influencers in your space attend your virtual party where you are the host and leader of the entire show!

In this segment, I want to give you the framework to set up your first webinar. It's not hard, but it is different than your standard "teaching Powerpoint". There are some real subtleties that you must master if you want to sell from a webinar. Let's get started.

Action – Determine if have something to teach others. If you do, then webinars are for you!

Day 72 – Teaching Vs. Selling

The first major difference between teaching and selling is the desire you create. When I teach a class on let's say stroke, I have a very standard method for putting my Powerpoint together. I might start with a case study, and then delve into anatomy & physiology, make some points, provide an overview of care, the hospital course, prognosis and long term follow up.

This is a standard lecture for the healthcare system - whether it's medicine, nursing or physical therapy. The problem is - it's so boring and predictable. You don't get to the end of the lecture and people are begging you to continue or asking how they can buy your book to learn more or pay you to continue teaching.

If anything, they are silently begging you to stop. More than half the class is doodling or daydreaming, the other half might actually be asleep.

It doesn't have to be this way. Ever since starting my business and learning how to do selling webinars, I have actually changed my academic Powerpoints. Now I certainly do not sell anything to my students, but I do want them to be interested in what I'm saying. The way you get people interested in to keep them hooked on what you are saying. This is what I want to teach you and will teach you as we move forward.

Action – Analyze your teaching style. Are you boring, entertaining, somewhere in between?

Day 73 – The Slide Deck

One of the first changes I made in doing webinars was to change out my webinar deck templates. Yes Powerpoint has a nice selection of slide templates, but they are pretty standard and only a few of them worth using. You can certainly use them, it's not a make or break deal, but I did change to a custom built deck.

Now a custom built deck may run you $20, $50 or $100 depending on how custom you want to get. Or you can create your own custom deck for free on Canva.com.

Make sure you use your brand colors and fonts in your Powerpoint deck. This way all of your process will look incredibly professional.

If you go on Canva and check out the professional created Powerpoint slide decks they offer, take a look at how minimalistic they are. This is going to be another change you must make.

Please do not put a lot of words on your Powerpoint slides. In fact 65-80% of your Powerpoint should be pictures or videos. Yes I know that is a huge change, but think about it. How do you feel when someone puts up a Powerpoint slide like this:

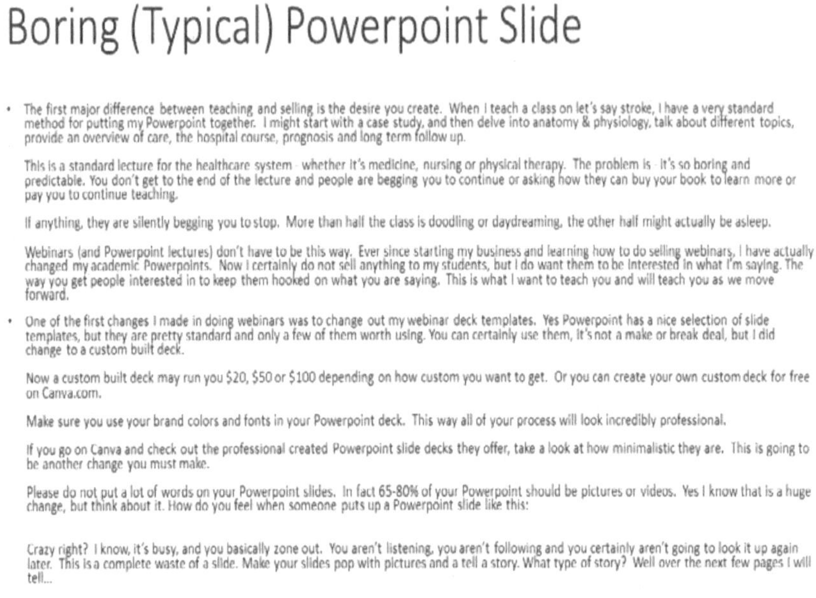

Crazy right? I know, it's busy, and you basically zone out. You aren't listening, you aren't following and you certainly aren't going to look it up again later. This is a complete waste of a slide. Make your slides pop with pictures and a tell a story. What type of story? Well over the next few pages I will tell you how to do it…

Action – Choose a slide deck to use with your branding colors and fonts. You can choose 3-5 different types of slide decks, but maintain the integrity of the branding.

Day 74 – The Webinar Story

To give a great webinar, the first step is to tell a story. The first step to a great story is the outline. There needs to be a beginning, a middle where something occurs and an end. Yes you must follow the standard path of story which is the beginning, conflict and resolution.

You can establish some kind of conflict in your webinar by providing case studies or talking about your own challenges.

Before you write out an outline of what your webinar will look like, you need to know what it's about.

What is the goal of the webinar? Are you selling a product or service? Are you establishing yourself as a leader in the field? Are you speaking for someone else? Is this a paid webinar or a free webinar?

Once you establish the goal of the webinar, then we can come up with a title. Your title of the webinar should be clear and NOT clever. Be very specific so you don't waste people's time. Attention is at a high premium. You don't want everyone, you only want your audience. So how could you title your webinar to entice your audience to come.

Let me give you a hint, it will not be: Major Cardiovascular Risk Factors In The Prevention of Ischemic Cerebrovascular Accidents. That is a super yawn, and I'm not sure who you would even attract with this title other than some neuro nerds.
Now if your audience was stroke patients, let's say you want to do some lifestyle coaching with them. You would definitely want to teach them cardiovascular risk factors, but you can't lead with that, because essentially no one will want to come. Instead your title could be: How John's 3 Simple Changes Saved Him From A Devastating Stroke - Again.

Isn't that at least more interesting? As a stroke patient, you know your recurrence rate is sky high. If you could make 3 simple changes and prevent a new stroke, would you at least want to know what they are?

Finally, which webinar seems more interesting?

Please note, the topic inside the webinar could be exactly the same, but if no one shows up, it won't matter what the webinar is about. Get butts in seats and then you can deliver your message.

Action – Create a headline based on who you audience is and then create an outline for the story.

Once you get people on your webinar, your next goal is to keep them there. If you start out dry and boring on your webinar, people will leave in the first 5 minutes. You need to edu-tain. A combo word educate and entertain. Now by entertain, I don't mean you have to act out or jump up and down, but you do need to maintain attention.

Think about how the movies do this. Most movies and stories follow a very limited number of plots. What they all tend to have in common is a beginning, middle and end. The beginning of a story is when we are introduced to the protagonist.

The protagonist is the hero of the journey. In a webinar you are NOT the protagonist. Contrary to what you might think, the audience needs to be the hero of the webinar. The hero in every story is flawed in some way. This creates the conflict.

If the story didn't have a flawed main character there would be no conflict and then there would be no story. It can't be that Mary does everything well, everything goes her way and now she is happy. That is a boring, horrible story. No, instead, Mary might be miserable, in pain, lonely.

Then something happens that changes everything and now she is happy.

The beginning of the story is you describing the state of Mary before the conflict. The first 5 slides need to be about the audience and what they are experiencing. You must empathize with their pains or struggles. When you talk to the audience where they are right now, you will capture their attention.

For instance, we just mentioned John and his simple steps to prevent recurrent stroke. If our audience is stroke survivors, then the story starts out describing John's first stroke and all the important struggles.

Action – Who is your audience and what are their current pains? Design 5 slides that describe the one thing your audience most struggles with.

Day 76 – The Conflict

Your role as the host is to describe either your audience's journey from pains and struggles or your own. Let's continue with our previous example. If you are a stroke survivor, you could describe your own pains and struggles from the stroke.

After you describe the "before", you have to create a climax point. Without a climax you have no story. For instance, Mary is miserable, then one day Mary woke up and she was happy. This is not only unbelievable, it's anti-climatic. It actually goes against the grain of human experience.

Something had to happen. What changed? Maybe Mary heard about new supplements or started an exercise program or found true love or found meditation elevated her to higher depths. Whatever it is, you need to describe the climax (conflict) in the next few slides.

Remember, use pictures to trigger your story to come out. You will need to practice several times to make sure the pictures trigger the right point that you want to convey.

The climax is the most important part of your story and should also relate back to whatever it is that you are selling. Don't tell a story about how Mary got happy using supplements when you are selling the idea of a keto diet.

You could say Mary's life changed when she made a simple change to her diet. Then ask the audience if they want to know what it is? They will likely be very interested to find out!

Action – What is the conflict in the story you are going to tell? Design 5 slides to show the conflict. Remember to use pictures and video (only a limited number of words)

Day 77 – The Teaching Chunks

When you are teaching in a webinar to sell, it's different than when you are teaching a class. Interestingly, teaching in a webinar is more exciting than the way we teach in a classroom and more effective. After you learn today's tip, you might consider utilizing this process whenever you teach.

Remember, you are always selling, whether you are "selling" products and services or you are "selling" a way of thinking, it's still the same method of influencing your listener. You must be interesting.

In a webinar, you want to reduce your message down to one main point that can be divided into 3 teaching chunks. Think about what you are talking about. For NursePreneurs, the main idea is to create a business. In order to help my audience understand how to start a business, I break the mega concept into 3 teaching points.

Does that mean that there are only 3 things to do to start a business? No, of course not. What it does is make starting a business seem possible. People will not do things willingly if they don't think it's easy or if they can do it.

Think about it. Have you ever been given the task of writing a 20-page paper? On the outset, it's a big deal right. What if I could break it down into 3 easy steps? Wouldn't that feel more doable?

In this case I would break the webinar down into: Teaching chunk #1 - Brainstorming the idea; Teaching chunk #2 Outlining the paper; and Teaching chunk #3 Drafting the paper. You are still writing a 20-page paper, but when you give the brain quick and easy wins, you are less likely to procrastinate and more likely to take action.

The teaching chunks are still pretty big ideas, so when you are teaching them, you break them down even further. Give your audience a quick win. What is one thing they can do quickly, easily and right away that will allow them to achieve something fast?

This works in the classroom and it works on a webinar. If they are successful in your quick win, they will want to know more and learn more from you.

The next part of the webinar is the MOST essential. Get this billion-dollar principle down and you will succeed every time.

Action – What is your main point of your webinar, what do you want your audience to walk away knowing? Then break down your main point into 3 (not 2, not 4, 5 or 6, just 3) teaching chunks.

Day 78 - Testimonials

Testimonials are called the billion-dollar principle because that is what they generate. Robert Cialdini eloquently discusses the power of social proof in his landmark book Influence. Think about any commercial or infomercial that you have ever seen (and bought from). The power of the commercial comes when normal, everyday people start talking about how the product or service worked for them.

The power of the testimonial is beyond compare. How do you use this in your webinar? You want to sprinkle the testimonials throughout. Any statement you make should be followed up with a testimonial that essentially echoes what you say. These testimonials can be written, in audio format or video which is most powerful.

The one place you must place your testimonial is after your teaching chunks. You want to teach 1 thing and then use a testimonial to show that it works. After my first teaching chunk - which is to help nurses see that they have an expertise, I have a student talk about how she became clear on her own idea of a business. After the second teaching chunk - which is how to accelerate success through setting milestones, I have another student talk about how easy it was to hit milestones in his business.

Now, a caveat - your testimonials must be real. Do not make up testimonials. This is not only unethical, it's illegal. The FTC spends its time cracking down on big names and big money, not small start ups, but all someone has to do is report you to send trouble your way.

The testimonial is powerful, make sure you use it ethically.

Don't have any testimonials for your webinar? Then get them. You shouldn't be teaching something that doesn't work or hasn't been shown to work.

Get a friend, a family member, anyone to use your product or service. You can even provide someone with your product or service for free in exchange for their honest thoughts.

Another great way to show something works is by using testimonials that other people have gotten. For instance, let's say you are teaching the keto diet.

There are lots of gurus who teach the keto diet – you can use quotes from them. There are also lots of people who have had success on the keto diet. If you find testimonials where the person says, the keto diet helped them lose 30 pounds, then use it.

Just be careful not to say that the testimonial is from working with you. The testimonial is simply that the keto diet works. There is a fine line here, so be careful!

A good number of testimonials to have is 5-7 preferably video, but written with a picture and a name works too. Use full names, not Sally from Kansas. Remember the testimonial has to be real.

Action – Collect 5-7 testimonials for your business.

Day 79 – Transition To Selling

After you are finished teaching your 3 points, your audience should be ready to hear more. If you have chosen the right audience and created desire with your teaching points, they will want to know how you have been able to achieve results.

For this transition, I simply let the audience know that I am going to reveal to them a process that has enabled me to live my life by design through a system that has taken me years to create and I will share it with them right then.

This is a smooth transition from teaching to selling. People will understand that you are now revealing a system that you have created. Some of your audience will jump off the webinar at this point. That is ok. Your webinar should be good enough to standalone. By this I mean, if you teach 3 points, someone watching the webinar should be able to achieve something by the end of your webinar.

If they want more, you offer more, if they have had enough, then you didn't waste their time. It's a win-win for everyone.

Use that transition, which will let your audience know the teaching is done and the rest of the webinar is letting them know how you achieved whatever results you did.

Action – Write out your transition sentence from teaching to selling

Day 80 – Academic Conferences

What if you want to use this methodology to teach but you are at an academic conference?

You can still use the same format of webinars in an academic conference. Obviously you will not use the transition to selling because that would be considered unethical to sell at an academic conference. In fact it would just be in poor taste to go on someone else's stage and sell anything without permission.

Make sure when you are presenting that you know exactly what you can and cannot do on stage or on a webinar. Selling would violate CE requirements in most cases.

So what can you do? You still provide the same value, keep the testimonials, because those are powerful.

You will end with some conclusions to your teaching points and let everyone know that there is so much more that you can teach them but you are simply out of time. If they want more information, please copy down your information and they should send you an email.

This way no violations occur, only people who are interested in learning more will contact you.

When those people email you, you can send them free gifts and training that you have already compiled and set them into your email funnel (remember we set up your email marketing system earlier in this book!).

Action – Tailor your webinar ending for academic conferences or "no selling" situations

ONLINE COURSES

Day 81 – Online Courses

Just to give you some bearings, we've gone over a lot of stuff in this book. I've shown you how to start a blog, set up a website, set up an email service provider, create your branding, how to start doing videos, get clients, establish your legal structure and do webinars. Now, I want to help you put together your online course.

Why?

Think of it this way, is there something that you explain over and over and over and over again? To the point that you are unconsciously competent in this topic? For me I tell nurses over and over again how they can leverage their expertise into a business model. I show them how to find ideas in my profitable idea blueprint course. This is an online course. It's relatively inexpensive and it provides coaching to those who take me up on the offer.

It took a little bit of effort to set up this course, but all the things I needed to set up the course were entirely free to me and they are free to you. In this segment of the book I want to show you how to easily set up your very first course.

Ready?

Action – Think of what a topic area that you could create a mini-course. Maybe your first course is 4 modules long. What is one major problem you could solve by teaching in 4 modules?

Day 82 – Remember The Audience

Before we can start putting your course package together, we need to know who we are speaking to. This is where you have to be absolutely clear about your audience. If your interest is chronic diseases, you need to find an angle where the audience will self-identify. What do I mean by this? Well chronic diseases could mean lyme disease, heart disease, diabetes, HIV, mental health, right?

You can't lump all these people together, your course would be all over the place. Think about it from the audience's perspective, if you had COPD, would you take a course that included people with lyme disease? It doesn't matter if the information is the same, it doesn't feel specific enough, so you have to be careful here.

Make sure your audience has a commonality amongst them, whether it's based on gender, race, demographics, age, disease, weight. If the group will self-identify then you can lump them together.

For instance, women over 50 living with chronic disease could work, though it's still a little vague. However, women over 50 living with lyme disease may be too narrow. It's important to find a sweet spot. You will narrow down your audience significantly and they may feel like you are speaking to them, but not so narrow that you are only speaking to a handful of people.

If you focus on lifestyle changes, you could do a course specifically for patients with chronic diseases, or you could create separate courses using the same material and specifically target heart disease and then modify it for diabetes, COPD, etc., though this could end up being a ton of work!

Action – For the next 24 hours think about exactly who your audience is and how do they self-identify? Then we can talk about what type of courses you can create.

Day 83 – Types Of Course Formats

What types of courses can you create? Well there are lots of options. You could have an e-book that sells for $49 if it truly has valuable information in it. If you take the e-book and add some videos and a workbook, you could easily sell that course for $99-297. (Remember I already showed you how to do videos earlier this summer!).

You could create a large course and sell it for $999. The higher in price you go, the fewer you will sell, so keep that in mind.

Sometimes it's good to have variable options for different types of people. Some people will just want the book, most people will want the middle of the road option and a few will want the most expensive thing you have to offer.

People learn in different ways. Some people will just want to read whatever it is you have to say. However, a lot of people will never read a single word you write. They will watch all your videos, so it's a good idea to teach in various different formats. I personally don't like watching videos, I want to read everything. Everyone will be different so it's nice to have different options available. In general, video has a higher perceived value, so even if you sit and read your e-book on video, you can charge more and you will appeal to more people.

If you absolutely hate the idea of being on video, you can record your voice over Powerpoint. Another free option is to simply load up your Powerpoint on Loom and record the entire presentation while you are speaking. You don't have to use a camera at all. It's still technically video.

Action – Decide what type of course format you will create.

Day 84 – What Do You Say?

What will you say or what will be on your Powerpoint?
When you present an online course, it can't be a bunch of word vomit. You don't just lay out everything you've ever learned about something on video. There is an art to teaching (refer back to the webinars section). The first thing you must know is that very little information can be absorbed at one time.

I know this is counterintuitive because when you were in school, they expected you to learn everything all at once. The fact is you retained very little what you learned in school (unless you have a photogenic memory). You really learned little by little with a lot of practice and reinforcement.

When you teach online, you can't teach too much. Otherwise you will shut your audience down. It's similar to our discharge instructions – Intensive Lifestyle Changes and follow up in the office in 6 weeks.

Don't make this mistake in your course. What could one person reasonably be able to accomplish in 6 weeks. How many changes can a person be expected to make without falling off the wagon?

You will need to go much more slowly than you think and break the course up into multiple courses if you need to.

Back to what to say on your course.

You may have heard about the teaching philosophy:

1. Tell them what you are going to say
2. Say it
3. Tell them what you said

You must follow this format, otherwise your audience will be completely lost. In fact at the end of every module you will need some sort of checklist that tells them in writing exactly what they learned. Otherwise your teaching is pointless.

I would add one more caveat here, don't provide 100% content. This will put your audience to sleep (remember being in class and your professor bored you to tears?). When you are selling an online course you must provide edu-tainment. You have to entertain your audience. Now this doesn't mean you tell jokes or jump up and down.

It simply means you need to add in stories, case studies and real emotion into your course to maintain attention. Imagine if your professors told you great stories during lectures that cemented the information they told you? In fact, I bet the only thing you remember from University are the stories you heard.

The formula is -- Content -- Compliance -- Emotion. Rinse and Repeat. Give your audience some solid content, make sure they are with you by asking if everyone is learning something (it doesn't matter if you are speaking to a computer screen, they will still perk up), and then tell a story. Go back into content -- compliance -- emotion.

Keep your videos short, less than 20-30 minutes. If you have a lot of content, break it up into a lot of videos.

Action – What is your teaching style and how can you teach your topic using the Content-Compliance-Emotion formula? Start gathering stories to tell.

Day 85 – How To Avoid Word Vomit

Ok, back to word vomit. One way to avoid this scenario is to flesh out your table of contents. How many main topics do you need to teach? Think about this one. How much information do they really need to know? What is the minimum amount that they need to know to make a change or see results?

You want to go for the minimum. In the case of behavioral change: less is more. This might be something that evolves over time. You might find that people need a little more info or a little less than what you offer, so then you just tweak your course.

For now we need to start with something, so let's say you are a diabetes coach. What does your client need to know? What are all the major problems that your clients have? List all the things you can think of.

Then group those things into categories. Ideally you will have maybe 5, 6, 9, 10,12 categories? Whatever it is doesn't matter, just as long as you hit all the things you need. Those categories become your modules. Each module is going to tackle 1 major problem.

You can have 4, 5, a zillion videos in your one module, whatever it takes to tackle that problem, but we need a limited number of modules. People need to think that they can accomplish your course and see results.

So no more than 12 modules. Ideally 6 modules, but this is strictly individualized and tailored to your audience, your preference and your situation. For a quickie course, 3 or 4 modules is sufficient.

Action – Make that table of contents of all the major categories you need to hit, then list the solution to those problems under the categories. These are the videos and teaching points you are going to need to make.

Day 86 – The Power Of Loom

For taking videos you really can't beat Loom (useloom.com). It's free and you can unlock all the features of Loom by sending an invite to 3 or 5 of your friends.

This will allow you to take unlimited videos for an unlimited amount of time. I actually just sent the referral link to 5 of my various emails because I was impatient. I am referring all of you, so I feel like I've more than made up for this "cheating" aspect of the process.

Once you unlock the powers of Loom, you can record just your desktop and present online lessons via Powerpoint, or you can have a recording of your Powerpoint with you at the bottom left of the screen so your audience can see you or you can just do a full on camera shot of you.

I've done all three and they work amazingly. All you need is your computer's camera and microphone. I think the sound is a little boxy on the computer, so I have a USB headset that I use to improve the sound, but if you don't want to spend any money, it's certainly not a requirement to have.

You can edit in Loom, but I find it cumbersome and prefer something else that I will tell you about, but if you really don't have a penny to spare, you can edit in Loom for free and then download a perfect mp4 video that can be upload directly to your courseboard or to your You Tube account, into Gmail or wherever...

I can't think of a single downside.. So you can get started right now. Start unlocking those features.

Action – Download a free copy of Loom and check out its features.

Day 87 – The Power Of Zoom

Now another great product I want to recommend is Zoom (zoom.us). I actually wrote a blog post on this that you can read here:

catieharris.com/using-zoom-interviews-in-your-nurse-business

so I don't want to spend too much time talking about how great this software is… But it is great, and it's free up to 40 minutes.

Action – Check out my blog post on Zoom: CatieHarris.com/using-zoom-interviews-in-your-nurse-business

Day 88 – Design For Your Course

Have you ever seen courses with beautiful Powerpoints and PDF graphics and great logos and such?

If you have ever looked into hiring a graphic designer you know that it costs a LOT of money! I'm hear to tell you it doesn't have to. Canva.com is a dream come true for anyone who has zero creative design in their body like myself.

You can create your own professional and unique Powerpoint slides in canva! Imagine your course having your unique logo, colors and design.

All I have to say is check it out. It's free. It changed my life. It saved me thousands of dollars and it made me look professional. Can you give a better rave review than that?

Action – Go check out Canva now. Make your logo, branding and first signature PDF.

Day 89 – Editing Your Course

Movavi is a video editing tool. It's more than that, it also is an audio editing tool and a screen shot tool and a recording studio.

Word of warning - you need a PC to use this effectively. I actually went out and bought a PC just to use it.

I explained this software when we talked about video marketing, I just want to re-emphasize it here. If you do any editing on video, this is worth the $75 bucks it costs. Check out my post on Movavi:

Catieharris.com/movavi-for-video-editing-is-king/

Action – Read this blog post I wrote on Movavi: Catieharris.com/movavi-for-video-editing-is-king/

Day 90 – Course Platforms

Finally, you have your system laid out, your Powerpoint slides created your videos done, you need to house them somewhere. Right? I mean how do people access them and pay for them? Well you have a couple options.

If you are eating spam out of a can and ramen noodles, you can set up a course for free on Thinkific. It's easy, and it's free, but it is also very limited. They will tease you with all the things you could do if you would just pay the monthly price. If you can resist that, then this is a great platform.

If you have a Wordpress website, you can set up Wishlist. Wishlist is a password protected course platform that will allow you to beautifully set up your course for a one-time fee of $169. It's lifetime access to your course board and I believe you can have unlimited number of courses on Wishlist, whereas something like Kajabi, which costs $129 a month will only allow you have 5 courses offered at a time.

Now another almost free option for delivering courses is using your You Tube account to host your videos (remember to set the videos to unlisted so no one can find them without your link).

You can then set up your Email Service provider, such as Active Campaign (remember when we talked about this earlier?) to automatically send your audience links to the videos and all the course materials based on when you want them to receive it. An email service provider like Active Campaign will cost you $9 a month.

Can you imagine the entire overhead of your business is literally $9/month? Everything else I've taught you in this segment was completely free.

So now the question is, what is stopping you from setting up a course?

If you are thinking, "who would pay to learn from me?" I can assure you, as evidenced by the billions of dollars spent on online courses, you could find 100 people to spend $97 on your course - that's almost $10k, better than any overtime you could do in a year.

Action – Choose the platform you want to host your course.

THE BOOK WITHIN

Day 91 – The Book From Within

Have you ever thought of writing a book? Maybe you think you will write the book once "something" happens in your life or your business or once you "make it", whatever that means.

I encourage everyone to write a book. Everyone has a book within them.

It's not hard, it's not rocket science and it's a guaranteed publication that gives you instant credibility. Think about it, any time you see that someone has a book, you assume they are an authority.

You can have this same instant success. And best of all, it's completely free!

In this final segment of 100 Days Of Action, I will go through how to write your book and get it published. I will teach you literally how to get it done in a weekend. It's fast, it's easy, and it's free.

What could be better? The only thing you need to do is to decide which book you want to write first.

Action – Make a list of all the book ideas you have.

Day 92 – Your First Book

The first thing you need to do in order to write a book is change your mindset. Your first book does not need to be a New York Times bestseller. It doesn't need to come out with any fanfare. It doesn't need to be a Random House publication. It just needs to exist.

The first thing you need to commit to is actually writing the darn thing. After you commit to that, then we can ask questions such as:

What are you going to talk about?

How long does this book need to be?

Where do I start?

To maximize your time and effort, I would use your first writing opportunity to talk about what your business is or what you want your business to be. For instance, my student Lori teaches DNP students how to write scholarly papers. She could write a book on how to write scholarly papers. Obviously right?

The same should be obvious for you. I wrote my first book NursePreneurs, on becoming a NursePreneur. Mallory Buxton wrote her first book on starting a Concierge Nurse Business.

None of these books make any money and they are not contenders for book of the year, but they serve a very important purpose. They get our names out there. My books for instance give me incredible SEO, and I can hold them up anywhere and people are impressed.

I recently had the experience of a friend of mine who was impressed by the fact that I had a legitimate looking book that was published. She posted it all over social media and my friends and family were like, wow, you wrote a book? I was like what?? Are you serious? For years, my family and friends referred to my business as "my little project", but when they saw a book they were impressed. All it took was a book to impress. I can assure you none of them read it, they just like to tell other people about it. My dad says: "Yeah my daughter wrote a book" to all his golf buddies, and I am instantly legitimized. It's somewhat annoying, but highly effective.

You'll have a very similar experience as well.

The length of your book is irrelevant. If it's 50 pages, it's 50 pages. That's how long Mallory's book was, and it led me to her.

I would never have found her without her publication. She has literally changed my life!

Your little tiny book can have a similar experience. It's as long as it takes you to say what you want to say.

This is no longer school, you are now writing for you and your audience period. The point of the book is to establish you in the field. That's all. Remember it's not up for Book of the Year. It doesn't define who or what you are. It simply puts you in the game. Let's get started.

Action – Choose 1 on your book ideas to focus on for this segment.

Day 93 – Your Table Of Contents

Let's go back to what actually goes into the book. The first thing you want to do is establish your main purpose. What is your main message?

If you are a diabetes coach, your book may be about living a healthy life with diabetes. Now what I want you to do is to pick 10 problems your audience has that prevents them from living a healthy life with diabetes. Brainstorm it out and come up with 10-12 problems. These 10 problems are literally your table of contents.

You have 10 problems which is 10 chapters. Now all you need to do is decide what the solutions are to the 10 problems. Again brainstorm all the solutions you can to the problems.

Perhaps Chapter 1 is Understanding the Diagnosis of Diabetes. The implication here is that patients don't understand diabetes (the problem). The solution? You could tell stories of patients you've had and how you helped them to understand diabetes, maybe you bring in some anatomy and physiology or maybe you talk about research. However it is that you help people to understand what diabetes is, goes into this chapter.

This chapter could be 1 page, 5 pages, etc.. If you write 10 pages per chapter, and write 12 chapters, you have a 172 page book. Not bad right?

Just don't get hung up on a 172 page book. There is nothing wrong with a 50 page book. Don't get caught up in the numbers game. It's about having the book that is important. Period.

Action – Draft your table of contents.

Day 94 – Writing The Hard Way

There are a few ways to bang out this book for yourself. I've done it a couple ways, so I'll tell you the hard way now and the easy way after this.

The hard way to write the book is to list out all your chapter headings and all your subheadings (which are your solutions). Think of each subheading as a blog post.

If the problem is Understanding Diabetes, what are 5-10 blog posts that you could write on this topic? Then write 1 blog post a day until that chapter is done.

For example

Chapter 1 – Understanding Diabetes

- What is diabetes
- Why is it a problem
- What are the consequences of uncontrolled diabetes
- What organ systems are affected
- Why most people don't manage their diabetes very well

This isn't actually a hard way to do it, but it's definitely an effort. I like to use a Google doc spreadsheet. I set up what chapters are going to be written, then add in the subheadings and finally put a date next to when that subheading (or blog post) needs to be written.

Remember to schedule or block off time in your calendar and verify that you actually have time on a particular date to write.

If you are skiing all day, you will likely not come back to the hotel and write a couple pages, so make sure you factor real time into your writing agenda.

Chapter 1 – Understanding Diabetes (complete by Jan 10)

- What is diabetes (1-2 pages completed by Jan 2)
- Why is it a problem (1-2 pages completed by Jan 3)
- What are the consequences of uncontrolled diabetes (1-2 pages completed by Jan 4)
- What organ systems are affected (1-2 pages completed by Jan 7)
- Why most people don't manage their diabetes very well (1-2 pages completed by Jan 9)

This way, I never have to "write a book", I just have to write 1 blog post on my schedule and then I'm done with my book for the day. I bet you could commit to that!

I call this the hard way because you have a little planning to do, and then you have to sit down and write your blog post for the day. Doing it this way may take you a few weeks to get it done if you are only doing 1 blog post a day or every couple of days.

Action – Map out how long it would take you to write your book this way.

Day 95 – Writing The Easy Way

There is an even easier way to get your book written, or maybe it's just faster. If you can talk more readily than talk your book out. There is no rule that the book has to be literally written or typed by you. You just need to provide the content.

You can use Google docs with a voice over recorder. Google will literally transcribe what you are saying for free. You can also record yourself talking and then send it to a transcriber. It's not expensive, maybe a dollar a page. If it's the only way you will get your book written it's totally worth the cost.

Another super simple way I've written books is simply to interview other people. I set up a call on zoom, record it and transcribe it. Do 10 interviews, add in an introduction/conclusion, a few aphorisms and boom! The book is completed.

It really can be this simple. Stop making it so difficult for yourself. The book is super important and it's a huge marketing tool, so get it done. Do it this weekend.

Action – Map out how long it would take you to write your book this way.

Day 96 – Repurpose, Repurpose And Repurpose

Now if you think of your chapters as a compilation of blog posts, then you should repurpose them. Before you publish, send some of your blog posts out as guest posts, put them on your own website, make videos of the topic, interview an influencer on the topic you are writing about. You could easily come up with 5 different ways to purpose every single blog post you write as a subheading for your chapters. Your book can also be multimedia.

Think about it, what if you write a solution as a blog post, then interview someone on the topic, add a QR code (which are free, just Google QR codes) to the book that links to that interview. There are so many things you could do. You can even generate traffic to your website with all this repurposing.

Use your book as an ethical bribe.

Tell people about a great download you have that people can access on your website. I hope you can see why the book is more than just a book. Remember the goal isn't to make money off the book, the goal is to establish yourself and generate marketing for yourself.

You can certainly post your entire book broken down into blog posts on your website. Don't stop there. Make those videos to post on YouTube or Facebook or Instagram. Map out what you are going to do. And guess what, if you miss an opportunity with this book, then you just need to write another one. Not a big deal!

Action – Plan out your repurposing plan. How many social media sites are you going to repurpose this content and when?

Day 97 – Self-Publishing

Once you complete your book, then all you need to do is self-publish it. This process is completely free. The best thing to do is to go onto Createspace. There are certainly other self-publishing sites that may be better, but they aren't free. For your first book, keep it simple and free.

Createspace is the self-publishing platform for Amazon. You can publish your book and it will print on demand when someone orders it. You then receive a royalty from Amazon without having to do anything else.

Createspace will manage everything after you upload the book.
I have a few books listed for $14.95. When someone orders my book, Amazon sends a request to print the book on demand to Createspace and then it gets shipped to the buyer. I don't deal with any of this. Amazon then sends me $6 in royalty payments.

It's great! You can even get a free ISBN code from Createspace. Talking about the pros and cons of paying for your own ISBN codes is really a conversation that is for your 2nd, 3rd or 4th book. For your first book, make all the mistakes, it's ok, just get it done.

Action – Check out Createspace and create an account.

Day 98 – Book Publishing Formatting Guides

Another great thing that Createspace does for you is provide you with formatting documents. I have a student Lindsay who created coloring books and she literally went through a ton of painful experiences in sorting this out.

There really aren't formatting guides for coloring books. If you have a complex book for some reason like Lindsay, I would strongly recommend you go on Fiverr and pay someone to format your book. It will save you hours of your life and tons of tears.

For everyone else who has a straightforward text, just download the Word template from Createspace. In fact, you might even start with the Word template and just write your book in the proper formatting in the first place. I personally like to work in Google docs, so this is not my preferred way, but you are not beholden to what I do. Do what makes sense for you.

Be sure to pick the size book you want first. The standard paperback is 6x9. I like the 7x10 books better. I used them for my journals and I use larger font than standard, so this size makes sense for me. However my book Nurse2NursePreneur is a 6x9 paperback.

Clearly the smaller the book size, the more pages there will be, so if that is an issue for you, then use the 6x9 format.

Action – Choose the size book you want and then download a preformatted Word template from Createspace so you can format your book properly as you write it. This will save you headaches.

Day 99 – Book Covers

Give your book a benefit driven title, such as: Break Free Of Diabetes Medications or Eat More With Diabetes.

Test out different names, ask friends and family which name is more appealing.

The title is important.

You wouldn't pick up a book that was called Excerpts From The Diabetes Counsel On Intensive Lifestyle Changes even if it were potentially life altering, would you?

Action – Give your book a title

Day 100 – Your Finished Product

The final piece to publishing your work of art is the cover! Createspace has a cover creator that you can use, and honestly if you want to get this done quickly and easily then just use it. If you are up for a little bit more of a challenge, you can create your own cover on canva for free.

Make sure you create the front and back cover on the PDF and include the spine. You need to account for the bleed as well, which is how the color runs off the book cover. Createspace will give you the dimensions to work in.

If you want to make your life super easy, then just get someone on Fiverr.com to create and format your cover. This may cost you $10-15. Don't waste your time and energy trying to make the perfect cover.

Use the back cover wisely. Do not leave it blank. Put a picture of yourself on there, add some information about yourself and put your website address on the back.

Remember, this isn't about selling your book and making passive income. It's all about marketing.

So get the word out! Give your book to family and friends. In fact, I would encourage you to order a bunch of copies and hand them out for free. Any time you meet someone who is your audience, imagine if you gave them a free book!

Everyone loves a free book. Unlike your business card, which they will throw out, they will keep the book on their shelves, on their tables and at top of mind.

Action – Create the front and back cover. Publish.

CONCLUSION

That's it you did it! 100 Days or 100 Minutes if you just skimmed through the book. That's ok if you did. You still have the blueprint to make it work. And heck if it takes you 100 weeks to get through the material, it's all good.

Remember starting a business, any kind of business is work, it's an investment.

I had a friend once who called me in a panic. Her boyfriend was about to start medical school and he needed money fast. She wanted to know what kind of business he could start on the side that wouldn't take up much time.

Really? I told her he should get a side job somewhere. Starting a business isn't like turning on a water faucet. You don't decide to start a business and then the money just starts pouring in. You have to have an idea, you need an audience and you need some persistence to get the two to match. When you get a match, then you can create a business.

Business is for creative people, people who want to help others and people who want to share something with the world. At least, the businesses that I start and help my nurses to start are based on this concept. Get rich quick schemes, well let's say the only ones who get rich quick are the ones making all the promises.

Business is about building a dream, your dream and seeing it realized. I hope this book helps put you in the right direction and the right mindset to get started. Remember the first year of your business is about learning, so take the pressure off yourself and just absorb everything you can.

Start putting the pieces together slowly and know that you are creating your very own destiny in the process.

Good luck and keep in touch with your success!

Catie

ABOUT THE AUTHOR

Catie Harris, PhD, MBA, and Registered Nurse is the NursePreneur Mentor who has empowered hundreds of nurses to monetize their knowledge and skills in business, while inspiring them to change the way healthcare is perceived and delivered. She strives to undo the perception that nursing care is limited to the hospital setting. Through her intensive mentorship program, Catie shows nurses how their nursing knowledge can transcend the hospital system into a profitable business.

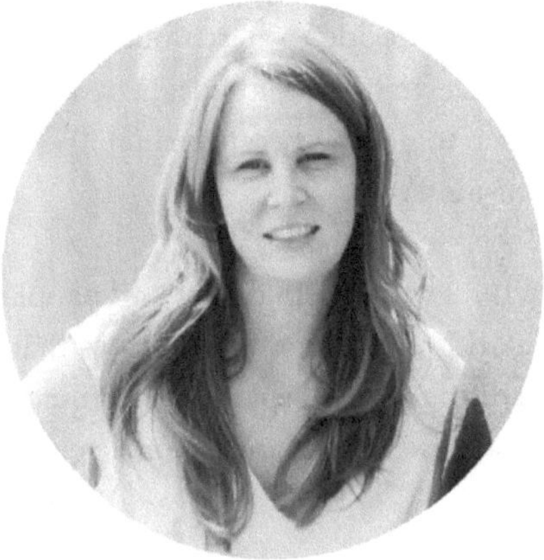

Catie mentors through one-on-one coaching, live events and her signature yearlong mentoring program: the NursePreneur Business Academy which can be found at www.CatieHarris.com/training

Catie is an international speaker who has been featured in ABC, CBS, NBC, Fox News and Huffington Post. She has also shared her innovative mentorship work on National and International Podcasts and TV including Be Efficient TV, Dubai One and Copy Chief with Kevin Rogers.

Catie is a serial NursePreneur (The NP Life, NursePreneurs, Concierge Nurse Services, Hydration Operation) and single mom living in Philadelphia with her son Matthew.

You can visit Catie on her website: www.CatieHarris.com

AND

You can follow Catie on Social Media:

Facebook: www.Facebook.com/nursepreneurs1

Instagram: www.Instagram.com/nurse_preneur

LinkedIn: www.LinkedIn.com/in/catieharris99

Made in United States
Troutdale, OR
11/03/2026

56852526R00086